J. L. Encarnação J. D. Foley (Eds.)

Multimedia

System Architectures and Applications

With 61 Figures

Springer-Verlag
Berlin Heidelberg New York
London Paris Tokyo
Hong Kong Barcelona
Budapest

Editors

José L. Encarnação
Fachbereich Informatik
TH Darmstadt
Wilhelminenstraße 7
D-64283 Darmstadt, Germany

James Foley
Georgia Institute of Technology Center
Atlanta, Georgia 30332-0280, USA

ISBN 3-540-57413-1 Springer-Verlag Berlin Heidelberg New York
ISBN 0-387-57413-1 Springer-Verlag New York Berlin Heidelberg

Library of Congress Cataloging-in-Publication Data.
Multimedia: system architectures and applications/J. L. Encarnação, J. D. Foley, eds. p. cm. – (Computer graphics, systems and applications)
Includes bibliographical references.
ISBN 3-540-57413-1. – ISBN 0-387-57413-1 (U.S.)
1. Multimedia systems. I. Encarnação, José Luis. II. Foley, James D., 1942- . III. Series: Symbolic computation. Computer graphics–systems and appli. QA76.575.M847 1994 006.6–dc20 94-14719 CIP

Printed in Germany

Cover Design: Konzept & Design, Ilvesheim
Typesetting: Camera-ready by authors
SPIN: 10085002 33/3140 - 5 4 3 2 1 0 - Printed on acid-free paper

Contents

Introduction

José Encarnação[1] and Jim Foley[2]
[1]Fachbereich Informatik, Technische Hochschule Darmstadt,
Wilhelminenstraße 7, 64283 Darmstadt, Germany
[2]Graphics, Visualization & Usability Center, Georgia Institute of Technology,
Atlanta, Georgia 30332-0280, USA

Multimedia computing represents the logical next step in the relentless march by which computing technology is becoming ever more useful and ubiquitous in our everyday lives. The first small steps were made by time-sharing systems. Next came interactive computer graphics and the graphical user interfaces developed at Xerox PARC and subsequently popularized, first by Apple and then by Microsoft and workstation manufacturers such as Apollo, DEC, HP, IBM, Silicon Graphics, and Sun.

Multimedia computing includes interactive computer graphics and graphical user interfaces, but is much more as well. First and foremost, multimedia computing concerns computer-based systems which create, process, present, store and communicate information in multiple representations, or media. Today, the representations are primarily visual and auditory. In the longer term, we can expect to see today's multimedia systems augmented by the force, texture, shape, kinaesthetic and olfactory feedback being explored in the context of virtual environments.

The visual media types of multimedia are text, graphics, and images. Text is of course a visual encoding of a language, while graphics includes either static or dynamic computer-generated material, which may vary in complexity from simple line drawings to photo-realistic renderings of highly-detailed environments. Images, in contrast to being synthesized, include digitized real world scenes, either static or dynamic. These are often called pictures and video, respectively. Text is of course just a special case of graphics: both text and graphics are computer-generated from models stored within the computer (the model may be as simple as a string of ASCII text or as complex as a solid model representation of a building or a city). Images, in contrast, are generated from the real world and do not have a model other than the bit maps which represent them (in some cases a model may be derived from the image).

The auditory media types of multimedia are speech, music, and sounds. Speech is an auditory encoding of a verbal communication language, while music is an auditory encoding of a structured notational system. Sounds, in contrast, are arbitrary and do not generally map to some model. Speech and music are to sounds as text and graphics are to images.

Of all these media types, it is the continuous, time-dependent media of audio, dynamic graphics, and video which taken together define the difference between the interactive computer graphics and graphical user interface technologies of today and the multimedia interfaces of tomorrow. Audio, dynamic graphics, and video are all relatively new to the computing domain, and they present new technical challenges and opportunities for dramatic improvement in our interactive systems.

From the perspective of technical challenges, multimedia affects nearly every aspect of computer hardware and software. Operating system scheduling must take into account the hard deadlines and synchronization required to play back a video with a sound track, or to keep a process visualization synchronized with a video playback of the actual process being controlled. Disks and disk farms must be organized to provide higher transfer rates than in the past, and to support multiple simultaneous I/O streams such as will be needed by video servers. Data base management systems require additional data types, new caching strategies to handle the massive size of compressed video files, new indexing schemes to access information based on visual or temporal characteristics. Networks need to be able to guarantee minimal levels of performance, degrade gracefully, offer both packet-switched and semi-permanent routing, mix together high bandwidth and low bandwidth traffic, and provide both point to point as well as broadcast services.

Hypermedia systems will need browsing metaphors to allow exploration of multimedia information. Graphical user interface development tools will have to accommodate the new multimedia data types, and at the same time offer advice to interface designers as to the most effective media in which to present different classes of information. Multimedia authoring systems may well merge with user interface development tools, but will certainly have to be more user- and task-oriented than presently in order to decrease the tremendous cost of preparing multimedia material (costs of 500 to 1000 person hours per one hour of multimedia material are not at all unusual!).

From the perspectives of improving our interactive systems, and perhaps more importantly, creating new classes of interactive applications, multimedia is exciting and important because it offers more engaging and productive interaction with computers. For instance, numerous studies have demonstrated that students learn more effectively with multimedia educational systems than with unimedia systems, because individual differences in learning styles are accommodated by the multiple media types, especially when the same information is presented in multiple media, such as text, images, and speech. To appreciate the power of multimedia, consider what a textbook or magazine or newspaper without pictures would be like, and whether you would prefer them with or without pictures!

The possibility of new classes of interactive applications is the most fundamental promise of multimedia computing. The long-heralded and now-occurring marriage of computing, communications, and information services is manifesting itself in literally dozens of new alliances between companies ranging from semiconductors to cable TV to newspapers to telephone companies to computer hardware and computer software. What was once the "battle for the desktop" of workstation and PC vendors fighting for control of white-collar workers' desktops is evolving into the "battle for the TV top" over who will control home-oriented multimedia and communications services. The types of services promised are many, and too long to enumerate here. The standard ones include video dial-tone, home shopping, interactive TV, integrated yellow pages and classified ads, integrated cable TV controllers and computers and home management systems, on-line multimedia libraries, and on and on.

The purpose of this workshop was to bring together a small group of multimedia computing researchers who would on the one hand identify research issues and agendas and on the other hand report on current research.

The workshop participants were:

Jerker Andersson: Infologics AB, Sollentuna, Sweden.

Friedrich Augenstein: Institut für Informatik, Universität Freiburg, Germany.

Jay Bolter: School of Literature, Communications and Culture; Graphics, Visualization & Usability Center; and College of Computing, Georgia Institute of Technology, Atlanta, Georgia, USA.

Martin Brenner: Abt. ZFE ST SN 71, Siemens AG, Munich, Germany.

Victoria Burrill: Informatics Department, Rutherford Appleton Lab, Chilton, Didcot, United Kingdom.

José Encarnação: Fraunhofer-Institut für Graphische Datenverarbeitung; Fachbereich Informatik der TH Darmstadt; Zentrum für Graphische Datenverarbeitung, Darmstadt, Germany (workshop co-chair).

Jim Foley: Graphics, Visualization & Usability Center; College of Computing; and School of Electrical Engineering, Georgia Institute of Technology, Atlanta, Georgia, USA (workshop co-chair).

Martin Frühauf: Zentrum für Graphische Datenverarbeitung, Darmstadt, Germany.

Bernd Girod: Kunsthochschule für Medien Köln, Cologne, Germany.

Ralf Herrtwich: IBM European Networking Center, Heidelberg, Germany.

Wolfgang Herzner: Hauptabteilung Informationstechnik, Forschungszentrum Seibersdorf, Austria.

Rainer Hofmann: KPMG Unternehmensberatung GmbH, Frankfurt, Germany.

Christoph Hornung: Fraunhofer-Institut für Graphische Datenverarbeitung, Darmstadt, Germany.

Wolfgang Hübner: Roland Berger & Partner, Frankfurt, Germany.

Takahiko Kamae: Hewlett-Packard Laboratories Japan, Kawasaki-shi, Japan.

Ken Knoespel: School of Literature, Communications and Culture; and Graphics, Visualization & Usability Center, Georgia Institute of Technology, Atlanta, Georgia.

Klaus Meyer-Wegener: Fakultät Informatik, Technische Universität Dresden, Germany.

Max Mühlhäuser: Institut für Telematik, Universität Karlsruhe, Germany.

Meinrad Niemöller: Abt. ZFE ST SN 75, Siemens AG, Munich, Germany.

Stefan Noll: Fraunhofer-Institut für Graphische Datenverarbeitung, Darmstadt, Germany.

Scott Owen: Hypermedia and Visualization Laboratory, Department of Mathematics and Computer Science, Georgia State University, Atlanta, Georgia, USA.

Ralf Steinmetz: IBM European Networking Center, Heidelberg, Germany.

Bernhard Tritsch: Fraunhofer-Institut für Graphische Datenverarbeitung, Darmstadt, Germany.

Kaisa Väänänen: Zentrum für Graphische Datenverarbeitung, Darmstadt, Germany.

Ana Sofia Vieira: Departamento de Matemática, Universidade de Coimbra, Portugal.

Frank Weller: FB Informatik, AG Hagen, Universität Kaiserslautern, Germany.

The material in this book is organized into three sections. The first section contains the reports of the three working groups, formed during the workshop, based on shared interests of the participants. The working groups are: Authoring Systems, Multimedia Systems Architectures, and Digital Video in Multimedia Systems. The following two sections are collections of related papers.

The first collection of papers concerns system architecture issues, and focuses on internal system matters such as multimedia data bases and networking support for multimedia. These papers include:

Tritsch and Hornung, "Co-operative Multimedia on Heterogeneous Platforms."

Herrtwich, "Distributed Multimedia Solutions from the HeiProjects."

Meyer-Wegener, "Database Management for Multimedia Applications."

Hofmann and Strack, "Towards the Modelling of Multimedia Environments: From the Image/Audio Signals to the Documents."

Girod, "Integration of Motion Video into Multimedia Computers."

Mühlhäuser, "A Modeling/Programming Framework for Large Media-Integrated Applications."

Steinmetz, "The Next Generation of Distributed Multimedia Systems."

The second collection of papers concerns multimedia documents and interfaces.These papers include:

Herzner, "Finegrained Synchronisation in Dynamic Documents."

Brenner, "Designing Multimedia User Interfaces by Direct Composition."

Andersson, "Using Conceptual Maps in Hypermedia."

Bolter and Knoespel, "Word and Image in Multimedia."

Working papers presented at the workshop were subsequently reviewed by workshop participants and by the following additional reviewers, whom we thank for their assistance with this project:

Mostafa Ammar, College of Computing, Georgia Institute of Technology, Atlanta, Georgia, USA

Wilhelm Barth, Institut für Praktische Informatik, TU Wien, Vienna, Austria

Peter Baumann, Softlab GmbH, Munich, Germany

Klaus Böhm, Zentrum für Graphische Datenverarbeitung, Darmstadt, Germany

Keith Edwards, Graphics, Visualization & Usability Center and College of Computing, Georgia Institute of Technology, Atlanta, Georgia, USA

Steven Feiner, Department of Computer Science, Columbia University, New York, New York, USA

Dieter Fellner, Institut für Informatik III, Universität Bonn, Germany

Ed Fox, Department of Computer Science, Virginia Polytechnic University, Blacksburg, Virginia, USA

Norbert Gerfelder, Fraunhofer-Institut für Graphische Datenverarbeitung, Darmstadt, Germany

Michael Gervautz, Institut für Computergraphik, TU Wien, Vienna, Austria

Hans Hagen, Fachbereich Informatik, Universität Kaiserslautern, Germany

Ralph Hill, Bellcore, Morristown, New Jersey, USA

Larry Hodges, Graphics, Visualization & Usability Center and College of Computing, Georgia Institute of Technology, Atlanta, Georgia, USA

Laurie Hodges, Georgia Tech Research Institute and Graphics, Visualization & Usability Center, Atlanta, Georgia, USA

Scott Hudson, Graphics, Visualization & Usability Center and College of Computing, Georgia Institute of Technology, Atlanta, Georgia, USA

Thomas Kirste, Zentrum für Graphische Datenverarbeitung, Darmstadt, Germany

Leszek Kotsch, Digital Equipment GmbH, CEC Karlsruhe, Germany

Rolf Lindner, Fachbereich Informatik, TH Darmstadt, Germany

Mike McCracken, College of Computing, College of Computing, Georgia Institute of Technology, Atlanta, Georgia, USA

Greg McLaughlin, Sun Microsystems, Mountain View, California, USA

Brian Michon, Digital Equipment Corporation and Graphics, Visualization & Usability Center, Georgia Institute of Technology, Atlanta, Georgia, USA

Heinrich Müller, Fachbereich Informatik, Universität Dortmund, Germany

Sham Navathe, College of Computing, Georgia Institute of Technology, Atlanta, Georgia, USA

Radu Popescu-Zeletin, Fachbereich Informatik, TU Berlin, Germany

Holger Rath, Zentrum für Graphische Datenverarbeitung, Darmstadt, Germany

Johannes Röhrich, Fakultät für Mathematik und Informatik, Friedrich-Schiller-Universität Jena, Germany

Dieter Roller, Institut für Informatik, Universität Stuttgart, Germany

Veronika Samara, Intracom S.A., Peania, Attika, Greece

Adelino Santos, Fraunhofer-Institut für Graphische Datenverarbeitung, Darmstadt, Germany

Alfred Schmitt, Institut für Betriebs- und Dialogsysteme, Universität Karlsruhe, Germany

Jürgen Schönhut, Fraunhofer-Institut für Graphische Datenverarbeitung, Darmstadt, Germany

Hans-Peter Seidel, Institut für Mathematische Maschinen und Datenverarbeitung, Friedrich-Alexander-Universität Erlangen-Nürnberg, Erlangen, Germany

Harald Selzer, Fraunhofer-Institut für Graphische Datenverarbeitung, Darmstadt, Germany

Rüdiger Strack, Fraunhofer-Institut für Graphische Datenverarbeitung, Darmstadt, Germany

Wolfgang Straßer, Wilhelm-Schickard-Institut für Informatik, Universität Tübingen, Germany

Norbert Streitz, Gesellschaft für Mathematik und Datenverarbeitung, Darmstadt, Germany

Charles Wiecha, IBM T. J. Watson Research Labs, USA

Hans-Peter Wiedling, Zentrum für Graphische Datenverarbeitung, Darmstadt, Germany

Peter Wißkirchen, Gesellschaft für Mathematik und Datenverarbeitung, Sankt Augustin, Germany

After the reviewers provided many helpful remarks, the paper authors were responsible for integrating the remarks in their papers. The workshop organizers alone were responsible for selecting the strongest papers for publication in this volume. We hope that our readers are pleased with the results.

Recognizing that multimedia will present new research challenges for years to come, a second Dagstuhl Workshop is being organized for July 4-8, 1994 by Dr. Ralf Guido Herrtwich of the IBM European Networking Center, with assistance from the organizers of the first workshop.

First Section

Group I Report: Authoring Systems

Group I Members: G. Scott Owen (Chair), Victoria Burrill (Rapporteur), Jerker Andersson, Friedrich Augenstein, Jay Bolter, Wolfgang Hübner, Wolfgang Herzner, Kenneth Knoespel, Kaisa Väänänen, and Frank Weller

Introduction

The objective of this group was to discuss the User's and Author's views of multimedia (MM). Authors are the Information Providers, responsible for the content, creation and maintenance of the information base. Authors use the tools provided by the developers. Sometimes the author is the user, and the user the author, i.e., in some applications, the author and user are the same person; in others they are different. The author is the person developing the MM applications (NOT the person developing the toolkit). The user *uses* the MM system.

There are different types of author: (1) Producers generate the text, pictures, video, etc.; (2) Integrators define the underlying hyper structure. These two types of author may be one and the same person, or they may be different. A third type of author is the Trail Blazer who does not change the data but adds to it. But these are all very fuzzy and blurred categories.

The first thing we did was to restructure the set of keywords into the following categories (in priority order):

- Application areas
- User interface
- Information structure and change
- Authoring systems

In each major category we prioritized the set of keywords, added and deleted them as we felt necessary, and then discussed them. We left Authoring Systems to the last not because this is the least important topic but because the discussion of the first three topics would mandate the requirements for the Authoring Systems.

Application Areas

The first topic discussed was Application areas. We did not discuss these extensively but listed and categorized them by the role of author versus user and other relevant issues, e.g., systems for computer literates versus "walk up and use" naive users. In some systems there is overlap between the roles of author and user in that an author might create the original system and the users might be able to modify the system, either by adding annotations or by changing the web of hyperlinks. In other systems this would not be true.

Are there really any application domains? There are lots of MM systems but who really uses them? Does this depend solely on who has the money to spend on them? There should be a huge market. Maybe people do not really understand MM? Once they see one good application to which they can personally relate and/or use then they will believe in it. The problem is finding that application. What do we think the best/most important MM applications are?

The first category was "Information Providers," which are systems that provide general types of information, as opposed to systems, e.g., training systems, which are focused on a narrow topic. The first example of this type of system is a Kiosk. We defined a Kiosk as a simple information provider with a very easy to use interface and extremely simple selection interaction method, though not necessarily of a simple internal information structure. These are oriented towards use by the general public, i.e., a "walk up and use" type system. A very simple example might be a museum kiosk and more complex examples would be a system telling tourists how to get around a city (as in ShareME) or college students how to get around a university campus. In a kiosk the author is distinct from the user, i.e., the user does not modify the system in any way.

A kiosk system is one where (a) the user and author are totally separate; (b) has a relatively simple interface (that is probably physically easy to use); (c) is an information provider for the general public (this is a sweeping statement); (d) a system for which the answer to "What is this system for?" should be blatantly obvious; (e) the information is not modifiable by the users (but it may not necessarily be a static structure).

The word "kiosk" is a general term, subcategorized by tourist information systems, encyclopaedias, etc. There was some discussion of cultural differences over this word; in the USA a kiosk is a system that dispenses information in a public place, with very limited functionality and very limited purpose; in Germany a kiosk is thought of as being a more general information provider.

A more complex information provider system would be an encyclopaedia with a large set of knowledge and thus, a more complex hyperspace. In an encyclopaedia an author creates the system and users may annotate and/or modify the web of links. This could include both the addition and deletion of links.

Other application areas include the following:

- Training
- Education
- Entertainment
- On-line electronic manuals

The first three areas require more complex information such as time dependence; interaction is less generic. For these systems an author creates the system and users may or may not modify the system depending upon the application.

Another application area is in Multimedia Monitoring, Control, and Decision Support Systems, such as a medical database or industrial plant monitoring. These systems are categorized by being very dynamic and having realtime changes. For decision support systems the users typically put in the structure and information for the system. For process monitoring and control systems an author will create the view and the information may be automatically updated for the user (control room operator).

Another application is Multimedia Computer Supported Cooperative Work (CSCW) with issues of communication and information content and sharing. A final category is Multimedia Simulation.

User Interface Issues

Under User Interface we grouped the topics (in priority order):

1) User Interface (UI) metaphors
2) Navigation
3) Dimensionality (2D and 3D, VR)
4) Interactive methods
5) Personalization

We then discussed each of the above topics.

User Interface (UI) Metaphors

A metaphor is the representation of one type of object by an analogy with another type of object. In our usage it is the representation of some aspect of the user interface by an analogy to a familiar object. Metaphors can be subclassed into physical, social, abstract and others. Several types of UI metaphors were listed, the first of which was Visual Representation. Next was Spatial Representation. We decided that there were two different types of Spatial Representation, the first were metaphors which used physical or realworld things such as a desktop or trash can. The second type was abstract, for example, a graph or a tree. There were also control metaphors. An example of this would be a button for opening a text window for scrolling. Another example would be a representation of a VCR or cassette player for video or animation and audio.

Metaphors cost something. If you use one you are "buying into" the metaphor it represents together with lots of assumptions and implications about it. There are connotations as well as denotations. Metaphors encapsulate a story. When you adopt a metaphor you take the good parts as well as the problems so that certain expectations may be associated with the metaphor that the system might not meet.

If you are building a MM system, what metaphors do you need? Some authoring systems use a score (temporal layout), others a stage and cast. Should author and user metaphors be the same? For example the Microsoft-AVI system gives the author the choice of whether or not to give control to the user, i.e., the user can be presented with just a video clip and no control or the full AVI control window.

How ubiquitous is the VCR control metaphor? It also applies to audio cassettes. But what happens when DAT tapes come along? What is the metaphor for accessing the tape frame by frame? Text is editable, but video is not—this is a crucial difference. Without semantics you cannot edit video. With current metaphors for video there is no easy way to allow the user to access a frame by content. The ZGDV/RAL MOVie project is addressing this problem.

There are several traditional disciplines upon which we should draw in designing multimedia interfaces. These include: architecture, graphic design, typography, dramatic arts and scene design, industrial design, etc.

Navigation

The next topic was Navigation. The questions here were "Where am I?", "How do I get where I want to go?", "Where have I been?" (backtracking), strategies and exploration. We decided to look at tools for navigation and then strategies. The parameters of Navigation issues include: size of the information space, absolute and relative indications of space and of elements, and subsets of modes, i.e., different views.

We came up with a large set of possible navigation tools including the following:

- Conceptual Map
- Guided Tours
- History lists or maps
- Keyword search (content search, incorporating Booleans)
- Structured search
- Index
- Contents

- Hyperlinks
- Random tool
- (AI) Agents to find something interesting (active or passive)
- Human expert
- Audio/video/animation hyperlinks (annotation)
- Video/animation search tool (index, storyboard)

A question was what new tools does MM require, if any? How do we handle the temporal aspects such as reaction times for various events. Can we track recurrent themes? Can we use the dynamic characteristics of the data within the tool itself or are we forced to map to a spatial representation in order to control it? For example, deaf people run video tapes at extra speed—this works on a VCR, so it should in MM, too, if we are using the VCR metaphor.

Along with the discussion on tools was a discussion of possible strategies which included the following:

- Plan a path to a specific goal or neighborhood
- Get an overview (detailed or superficial, i.e., at or greater than the granularity of the information)
- Exploration
- Ask for help
- Serendipity

The first tool discussed was a Conceptual Map, which gives an overview of the hyperspace as either a textual view or a spatial representation. As a spatial representation this could be a 2 or 3D graph or tree, scrolling walls, rotating 3D trees, or a fish-eye view. The fish-eye view shows the neighborhood of the user in great detail, but areas farther away in less detail. The fish-eye view can be textual or it could be a spatial view of the conceptual map. For a fish eye view the relative "distance" between nodes must be known and so the concept of "distance" in the hyperspace must be defined in some manner.

Maps can be active navigation devices, or they can be passive aids to orientation. An active map would allow the user to immediately jump to any node by pointing to that node, i.e., it would be able to dynamically create a link between the present node and the desired node. This link could be temporary or permanent. A passive map would show the user a path, if one existed, from the present node to the desired node but would be incapable of creating any new links. There could also be a temporal map, for example: audio or music.

Another tool is a Guided Tour where the user follows a predetermined path. There might be several such guided tours, one for each set of users. This is one way to customize the system for different users. The user might be restricted to the Guided Tour or they might be able to leave it at any point to go on a side trip. Note that a restricted Guided Tour reduces hyperspace to a linear space.

Another tool is a History list (list of previously visited nodes) or map (the same information in map form). This allows the user to immediately return to any previously visited node. However, this list might grow very large so an alternative or companion tool would be Bookmarks which the user could use to mark a visited node for returning later. The Bookmark list would be much shorter than the History list.

There are several tools that can be used for queries, i.e., trying to find specific information. An Index or Table of Contents could be used for a topic search and a Keyword search, with Boolean operations, would be a content search. There could also be a structured search, for example "Show me nodes with certain characteristics." Hyperlinks themselves could be considered as tools to navigate Multimedia space. Another tool would be a Random Tool which would be "Take me anywhere but here." There might be a human expert available, via a network, such as in the ShareME system.

We also considered Artificial Intelligence-type agents. These might allow the user to say "Take me somewhere interesting." The user could possibly define "interesting" or the agent could have observed the user and take them to a place similar to previously visited nodes. Another tool would be audio/video/ animation hyperlinks and/or annotations such as MOVie. There might also be a video/animation search tool which might be an index or storyboard.

Strategies

We discussed strategies that could be used to plan a path to a specific node or to a neighborhood or else to just browse an area. We divided strategies into two categories: those which aimed at a specific goal and those in which the goal was non-specific or fuzzy. Some tools may be useful for one strategy; some for the other. We created a matrix of tools against strategies, which is shown below.

Tool\Strategy	Specific goal	Fuzzy goal	Exploration
Active Map	x	x	x
Passive Map	x	x	x
Guided Tour	--	x	x
History Lists	x	--	--
History Maps	x	x	?
TOC	--	x	--
Index	x	--	--
Content Search	x	x	--
Structure Search	?	x	--
Hyperlinks	x	x	x
Random	--	--	x
Agents	x	x	x

Specific goals	=	"I want this information" (a specific query)
Fuzzy goals	=	"I want something about..." (everything about a subject)
		- increasing desire for specificity -
Exploration	=	"What is here?" (general enquiry)

x = The navigation tool is useful in attaining this goal.
-- = The navigation tool is not useful in attaining this goal.
? = The navigation tool may or may not be useful in attaining this goal.

Other strategic possibilities include: ask for help, general overview, serendipity, and exploration. We also noted that there may be system (automatic) strategies as well as user's strategies. For example, the system can guide the user toward a specific goal.

Dimensionality Issues

There are at least four categories of dimensional representation for the user interface: 2D, projected 3D, true, stereoscopic 3D, and Virtual Reality. Each of these may be useful for some applications. It is a research question whether and when 3D interfaces are useful. Also we noted that one can use a 3D metaphor without true 3D display.

Interactive Methods

Here we noted two issues that are especially relevant for multimedia interfaces: temporal issues (dealing with the dynamic character of the information) and 3D representations. Again, 3D input devices (e.g., the data glove) are not necessarily required for 3D representations.

Personalization

In general, personalization methods may includes adding or deleting links, creating different views, macros, markings, including bookmarks, and annotations. Issues of particular importance to multimedia include speed of interaction and mapping among media. This latter is important, for example, for users with disabilities. Video is of no use to a blind user, so we might try to remap video information to the audio channel. Multimedia applications can also be personalized according to the different skills, interests, or knowledge level of the user.

There are new dimensions of time; the user may want to specify a preferred medium for reasons of personal preference or according to equipment available. This is especially important for visually challenged users. The mapping of one medium to another (or one medium to a different form of itself) is another interesting research area.

What forms of personalization are there?

(1) By content to reflect a person's interests, e.g., sports.
(2) By abilities to present the same information via different media according

to personal skills and/or the equipment available.

(3) By knowledge according to whether the user is a beginner or expert.

Information Structures

The integration of different media and/or importing devices defines a central purpose of information structures. Information structures create hierarchies that determine the levels that an author will be able to access and thus, place limits on the author. Such control determines the flexibility the author has of working within the system. Information structures also affect the way the information is presented to the user. Information structures are shaped not only by the media to be integrated but also by the psychosocial patterns that influence the way information is structured. The issues in information structures include the following:

- Granularity
- Restructuring of information
- Metainformation

Logical data models

Logical data models are paradigms or significant structures that determine the capabilities and possibilities that the author has in structuring information. Several categories of logical data models can be identified:

- Nodes and links
- Object Oriented structures
- Relational models
- Ordered sets
- Stacks (as in HyperCard—an example of an ordered set)
- Flow Charts which indicate progression plus synchronization (an authoring metaphor but not really a data model)

The first four categories were felt to be "serious" structure models whereas the last two were "toys." For example, while HyperCard itself can handle huge stacks the question is whether an author can control a large amount of information structured only by stacks.

One thing that all these models have in common is that they are discrete representations based on units of information and that they make use of methods of navigation and selection. There are various ways of defining nodes and links. Logical data models are comprised of a basic structural paradigm and well-defined information units. Information units can either be simple or compound. It is also important to recognize that information units can be realtime or continuous feeds.

Granularity

Granularity appears on different levels. While it may appear in hyperspace (granularity of information space) it is also a factor within one medium (granularity of medium). Granularity of medium has significant ramifications for the integration of different data types. The author potentially has access to any granularity, provided that it is supported by the authoring tools. The author may wish to limit the options available to the user. The granularities offered to the user determine (or, conversely, are limited by) the storage formats and realtime performance.

Restructuring of Information

Restructuring allows the user to modify the information space at hand. The question arises: Is it necessary to have access to the explicit structure in order for it to be modified? Annotation (making comments on a node or link) may, or may not, be an act of restructuring based on the logical model functionality. It may be an overlay or add-on or change the actual node and link structure. Annotations should be "hidden" from other users. Adding and deleting links assumes that the links are embedded in the information. Individual users may have their own webs. Annotations *may* be like a restructuring, but not necessarily.

The following questions arise:

1. What changes can readers make to the original information?
2. What is restructuring? Adding one node? Deleting one node? Adding an annotation? Can a user do these? Permanently? Probably "yes" to all but the last question.

Where is the boundary between adding and modifying the information? Providing that you can get back to the original then it is an add operation; if you lose the original then it is a restructuring. Restructuring might be defined as adding or deleting links. These are very low level operations. High level operations include adding links of a specific type to all nodes (such as adding help). So restructuring is determined by the underlying data types.

Both authors and users may add links, but this depends on the model. You may want to allow user modifications of the form "This link added by xyz." The user may be restricted in restructuring; the author should be able to do the major restructuring but what facilities does this involve? There are implications on the author who restructures since this may mean that user's links become invalid.

Restructuring makes the user become a co-author. What constitutes a restructuring is a research issue.

Metainformation

Metainformation is essential for some navigation tools and for complex restructuring operations. For example, the HyperCard model is implicit, so it is difficult to do large-scale restructuring. The storage of metainformation may be internal or external to the information space. We would notice that questions involving the storage of metainformation were not addressed. It is either associated with the information units and link structure or may be completely external to the information space. Metainformation may also be shaped by metaphor and may contain logical implications embedded within the discourse structures suggested by the metaphorical associations.

Authoring Systems

Editing in different media currently may involve several editors, translations, then final integration together. But this is a failing of current MM authoring systems which provide very few integration facilities.

Input and transformation of different media types should be transparent to the user. At the moment, different media types are integrated together via different tools, i.e., editors are medium-specific. We need a more document-oriented environment. It is more convenient for the author to have everything incorporated in the authoring tool. It is of course possible to prepare items outside the authoring system and then import them, but integration is better.

An authoring system is an environment with different tools for different tasks. Sometimes the author has to generate information, import it, modify it, restructure it, provide references to it (especially in a power station or other realtime application where data is constantly being generated), design/decide on the user interface, and then finally integrate it all (by setting up nodes and composing them). This process is subdivided by data types, and further complicated if the application is distributed. SGML can be used to define logical levels of information. Within composition, we also need a metaphor for successful integration.

MM Document Design

What guidelines should the author use? Guidelines are needed that do not overload any one human sense channel. These guidelines are for structuring information together. Should these guidelines be provided by the system? Written guidelines are often ignored. Some systems impose guidelines and accept that the resulting system is not 100% flexible, but this may be a necessary trade-off.

Guidance versus Flexibility

The system should monitor itself and warn the author if the guidelines are being ignored. An example would be grammar checkers and design advisors. The system could ask the author if they really want to do this. The system has *suggested* guidelines but not rigid rules.

A major question is what is good MM document design? Paper documents have standards developed over 400 years whereas MM standards are very young, and are still being developed. This is another good research area.

What language should the guidelines be in? This depends on the metaphor of the application, but how do we describe it? Would "Design Templates" be a better description of these guidelines?

The first thing we did was to define the authoring tasks as follows:

(1) Acquisition and generation of information:
- create information
- import information (file in, static images)
- reference to external information, dynamic
- edit information

(2) Choice of design metaphor

(3) Structuring of information:
- integrate information, e.g., set up nodes
- structurize information
- produce user interface, e.g., layout, colors, etc.

(4) Information and Structure Maintenance and Enhancement:
- update
- correct/repair
- ensure consistency
- restructuring

Several current problems were identified including the following:

(1) Authors use many different tools for completing the task.

(2) Authors tend to do bad document and application design.

(3) The quality or level of editing tools varies for different content classes, e.g., high for text and graphics, lower for images, and even lower for video and audio. Whereas text editors have had several generations for refinement, tools for the other media types are in their first or second generation.

(4) Few tools are available for integrating the different forms of information, e.g., the editing of different classes such as subtitling a film. This is a corollary of point (1). We also need a suitable format for accessing and synchronizing the media—this is a corollary of point (3).

(5) Current tools do not provide sufficient support for spatial or temporal dependencies, e.g., concurrency and synchronization.

(6) Metaphors. The use of multiple metaphors within one system are acceptable in order to achieve different results and granularity of design. The authoring tool should provide metaphors for the user interface, but the author should be able to select and refine these as required. We may require additional metaphors for the author and user, and correlation of metaphors. There needs to be consistent metaphors for authors.

(7) Authors are not usually experts in design or in computers so the authoring tool should be easy to use, e.g., ShareME. There is a trade-off between easy-to-use and low-level flexibility that a programmer should be able to handle. Can we layer the authoring system? We need layered tools with levels of capability and required expertise. Are templates useful for this? The author can use the templates as far as possible but the system should be extensible and allow the author to go beyond these if required.

(8) Ideally, we would like people or authors to be able to do everything, but the creation process will probably require a team of different experts for each of the different tasks. Traditional methods such as film making involve a vast number of different people for different tasks. Thus, we need tools for team development (both one site & distributed).

Tasks for the Future

(1) Authoring tools should provide a more integrated environment, and provide better integration together of the different media. We need authoring environments and not just authoring tools.

(2) The flexibility of existing tools is not that expressive for temporal and layout tasks, for example, the position of windows is often controlled by

the Window Manager. There should be improved placement controls for the author when positioning things in time and space.

(3) We need to find metaphors for authoring systems, and improve existing metaphors such as a script, score, or storyboard. We need to provide consistent metaphors or consistent interoperation between metaphors.

(4) We must improve content editing, both techniques and tools for image and video. An example is MOVie which provides a tool for mapping a screen area for video. We should move towards automatic video and image editing.

(5) We must provide the author with guidelines for good design, i.e., the authoring system should advise the author in the following:

- Selecting the most suitable metaphor
- Selecting the most suitable multimedia layout
- Creating a good structure

(6) What is a good multimedia layout? We need to learn from well established concepts, e.g., typography.

(7) We need to explore the mapping between different media, e.g., text to speech, video to VR, and mapping between different forms of the same media to allow for disabilities, personal preferences, skills, equipment, etc. Which mappings are sensible and which are the most effective? Can they be generated automatically?

(8) We need to provide additional specific components within the authoring systems to enable development of distributed MM applications. e.g., teleconferencing, distributed kiosks. There is a need for:

- Personalization (different user views for distributed information)
- Structuring distributed information
- Specific components within authoring systems to provide for this

(9) We need to provide tools for team development (cooperative authoring systems) or CSCW applied to MM authoring—both one site & distributed.

(10) We need to establish standards for structuring information and cooperative authoring, for example by improving SGML, ODA, HyTime, etc. Make sure these systems are robust enough to be able to cope with emerging solutions and techniques.

Group II Report: Multimedia Systems Architectures

Group II Members: Martin Brenner, Martin Frühauf, Christoph Hornung, Klaus Meyer-Wegener, Max Mühlhäuser, Bernhard Tritsch

Overview

The overall goal of this working group is to define a framework for multimedia architectures, and to state requirements for other groups (such as the work group 1 dealing with multimedia user interfaces). To reach this goal, it was decided to put several position statements together.

First, different views on architectures are presented. They define a multi-dimensional space, each dimension spanning a certain independent aspect. Outgoing from this space, different paths are elaborated in more detail, leading to different position statements. This is clearly not yet a well-defined architecture, but may rather be seen as a first sketch to gather information about what aspects have to be considered. One aspect considered in more detail is formed of the underlying information types, i.e., multimedia and cooperative access. First, a definition of the information type multimedia is given. Herewith, a clearer understanding of the underlying information is achieved, and requirements to other views are formulated. Multimedia is seen here in conjunction with Computer-Supported Cooperative Work (CSCW). This information type is explained next in more detail.

Orthogonal to this, some of the function categories are elaborated in more detail. Data management is concerned with the aspect of long-term archival storage of multimedia information. It thus has to cover device management, data type (schema) management, search facilities, transfer of large volumes of data under time constraints and compression techniques. Communications deal with the transfer of large volumes of multimedia data over various types of networks. Exchange of data has to be executed in realtime and isochronously, i.e., the elapsed time required to transfer a certain amount of data has to be predictable. The data transfer services should be fault-tolerant and reliable. Security aspects of data exchange in common networks have to be considered. At last, the aspect of application development has been considered. Tools are available and are continuously being improved to handle multimedia data. They must be integrated in a much smoother way than is the case today.

All in all, these are just different paths through the multidimensional architecture space. At some places, they meet—but it is just too early to combine them into a single architecture that covers all relevant aspects of multimedia systems.

1. Introduction

At the beginning of a discussion on multimedia (MM) system architectures, one cannot avoid the question: What is a multimedia system? This alone could be the subject of a fierceful debate. However, there are some proposals, and for the sake of brevity, they will be used without further questioning. In [Stei90a], Steinmetz, Rückert, and Racke suggest that "a multimedia system is characterized by the computer-controlled, integrated processing, storage, presentation, communication, creation, and manipulation of independent information that stems from several time-dependent and time-independent media" (p. 281).

The next question is just as difficult: What is an architecture? An architecture is a certain view of a system (or of large number of similar systems). It gives a comprehensive picture of either the functionality or the implementation of the system, leaving out the details, oversimplifying it to some extent, but making clear the main concepts, building blocks, and/or principles. Hence, an architecture can also be regarded a (complete) set of design principles: It simplifies the task of building a system, since it gives a gross structure and helps to remember all the subtasks that have to be accomplished.

An architecture should also provide a common frame for a variety of systems with different properties concerning performance, cost, etc. Applications will then select and tailor first the functions (services) required and then accordingly the building blocks. Tailoring can be as easy as setting a few parameters, but also as difficult as writing programs. This can be used to support:

- flexibility
- scalability
- interoperability
- quality
- reliability

Consequently, decompositions of existing multimedia systems should be guided by architectures, i.e., they help identify structure in those systems. Various aspects of the systems can be structured, e.g.

a) Structure the functionality w.r.t.
   - level of abstraction, i.e., the (virtual) objects manipulated

- level of integration (of media)
- contents, structure, and access (the CHM cube)
- the media

b) Structure the hardware:
- hardware/software boundary
- bottlenecks
- typical configurations: MPC ($5,000), MM workstation ($50,000)
- codecs
- network adapters

c) Structure the software:
- in layers
- in components
- according to functionality
- interfaces and protocols
- codecs

2. Views on Architectures

As we have seen, there is a common understanding that systems usually do not have a "single" architecture, but that different architectural views can be drawn, describing systems (and problem domains) from different perspectives. First, the following possible basic views on architectures have been identified:

- information types (access, structure, content)
- categories of functions/services
- hierarchy of services (interfaces)
- hardware/software distribution, configuration, service integration
- application integration

Second, it seems worthwhile to summarize possible "elements" which an architecture might be made of. Such enumerations of elements follows below:

- functions (services)
- building blocks (components)
- interfaces and protocols

Third, functions can be grouped with respect to certain application classes or complex interoperations of components, leading to:

a) A CSCW view of multimedia systems:
- concurrent access

- sharing of data and workspaces
- joint editing

b) A data management view of multimedia systems
- archiving functions
- representations = codings = formats
- types instead of formats, i.e., access functions (operators)
- application neutrality

c) A communications view of multimedia systems
- allocations of components to nodes
- client/server systems

d) An application developer's (programmer's, author's) view of multimedia systems
- tools, toolkits
- configurations

All these different aspects and views will be discussed in more detail in the following.

2.1. Basic Views

The basic views are seen to be independent of each other, herewith defining an n-dimensional space.

The information types distinguish between access, structure, and content information. Herewith, basic information entities are identified, out of which complex "documents" can be composed.

The function categories distinguish between processing, transfer/ communication, storage/retrieval, presentation, and interaction/capture. This view is based on "abstract devices" providing services.

A complex system consists of several service levels. Hardware, drivers, basic services, toolkits, and frameworks have been identified.

These services then must be mapped onto software and hardware components. This leads then to issues like configuration and service integration (not yet elaborated).

The view application integration deals with the integration of multimedia into applications. Here, the levels "single media," "integration to multimedia," and "media-integrated systems" have been identified.

2.1.1. Information Types. A central question when defining the architecture of an information processing system is the definition of the type of the underlying information. To avoid the confusion that often occurs with the misleading usage of the terms multimedia, hypermedia, or cooperative work, a distinction between the following information types has been made:

- access
- structure
- content

These information types are orthogonal to each other and form basic entities, out of which complex documents can be composed. Time-variance is another basic concept which can be applied to all the information types.

2.1.2. Function Categories. This view is based on abstract devices. They can be seen as abstractions of types of real hardware devices providing different kinds of services. The following function categories have been identified:

- processing
- transfer/communication
- storage/retrieval
- presentation
- interaction/capture

The separation of function categories allows the clear definition of basic services, out of which a hierarchy of services with increasing complexity can be built.

2.1.3. Hierarchy of Services. Different levels of abstraction may exist for these function categories; leading to the layering of a software architecture. A common view of such layering is as follows:

Device drivers: This level is not considered visible or important to the application user or programmer.

Basic services: Offered as part of the hardware/software platform (e.g., the operating system or the network services, see below); the interface is usually an API.

Toolkit functionality: These are application-independent functional blocks which often belong to one of the above-mentioned categories; they are often interfaced via APIs.

Platforms: On the same level, one may find what is sometimes called platforms. These are attempts to standardize a set of underlying functions in a domain-independent manner across heterogeneous underlying systems (i.e., media peripherals, computer architectures, or the like). Examples are Apple's QuickTime-based platform or Microsoft's Multimedia Workstation platform.

Frameworks: Combine several underlying functions and tailor them to the needs of an application-domain such as banking, CASE, computer-aided instruction, etc.

Application functionality: Off-the-shelf tools like authoring systems, or home-grown, i.e., customized or custom-built dedicated applications.

The above layers define a hierarchy, which also indicates a stepwise movement:

- from device-dependent to device-independent
- from generic (application-independent) to specific (application-dependent)

2.1.4. Hardware/Software Distribution, Configuration, Service Integration. This view deals with the integration of multimedia into applications. Here, the following levels have been identified:

- single media
- integration to multimedia
- media-integrated systems

2.1.5. Design Principles and Client/Server Considerations. While today client/server-based architectures are considered the state-of-the-art, they are in fact questionable. One might define three degrees of sophistication of distributed software architectures:

- Monolithic Systems
- Client/Server Systems
- Object Migration

The only distribution aspects of monolithic systems may stem from the capabilities to exchange files or information based on point-to-point user-invoked communication tools.

Client/server systems support distribution and stem from a scenario in which more and less powerful machines exist in a system, the less powerful ones being typically located at the users' sites. Client/server systems draw a lot of attention from the fact that they are mostly programmed based on the RPC (remote procedure call) paradigm, which is claimed to be "almost identical" to the well-known procedure calls in traditional programming.

The client/server concept has a number of drawbacks: First, the natural world is not separated into pure clients and pure servers; rather, most people act as clients and servers interleavingly. Real world modeling in software should allow to adapt to this. Second, since workstation power boosts, the distribution of powerful and less powerful machines may change rapidly in an organization, so the appropriateness of a system as client or server may change faster than the operators can cope with that change. Third, client/server software architectures draw—early in the lifecycle—a solid border line between client and server and define the protocol between them (cf. X Windows and the X-Windows protocol). Over the years, or even from one situation to the other, this borderline may turn out to be inappropriate, and the wish may arise to move this borderline, which is not possible in most systems.

Object-oriented distributed systems lead to a large number of fine-grained objects; their distribution among different workstations can be defined at startup time or even at runtime, if object migration is supported in the system. Moreover, the object-oriented approach supports the real-world modeling as requested above and is not bound to a strict separation of clients and servers.

2.2. Combining Different Views

The different views, when considered isolated, just allow to make rather general statements about the architecture of a multimedia system. However, by combining them, we get a narrower view to certain problems. As an example, the following refinement would be possible:

- multimedia information (definition of data types and methods)
- storage/retrieval of multimedia information (MM data bases)
- service hierarchy in MM data bases
- distributed MM data bases
- distributed MM data bases for banking applications

Please note that important areas such as operating system support and media processing support (cf. "software architecture" components as described in the chapter below) where not addressed due to time constraints and, in particular, due to the fact that no corresponding buzzwords were collected during the workshop.

3. Contents Information: Multiple Media

The first central point discussed in more detail was an attempt to define the characteristics of multiple media been the underlying contents information of a multimedia system. The different media types and their characteristics play the major role in a multimedia system.

3.1. Media Types

The usage of multiple media was seen as being essential to support both an almost natural human-machine interaction as well as an efficient computer support human to human communication. The latter one can be seen as the exchange of messages. Therefore, a first attempt was made to identify natural sending and receiving of information. In a multimedia system, sending is then realized via input devices, while the reception of messages is done via output devices. This leads to a scheme with the following keywords:

- Information Type: the human sense related with the exchanged information
- Devices: computer-supported input/output devices for information exchange
- Message Type: human interpretation of the exchanged information
- Multimedia Object: computerized representation of the exchanged information

3.2. Natural Human Media Resolution

In order to define the requirements of multimedia systems, the natural human media resolutions must be pointed out clearly. This includes both temporal and data resolution. The data resolution in bits refers to the amount of data necessary to store one sample of media information

The visual and audio information types ("See" and "Hear") are used for active communication ("Show" and "Say"), sometimes the tactile information type ("Feel") is included ("Touch"). Taste and Smell are almost always passive media.

The amount of data needed for the media is very high for the visual information type (> 1 MByte/sec.), moderate for audio (< 500 KBytes/sec.), and low for the tactile, tasty and smelly information type (< 1 KByte/sec.).

The constraints of a computer system that have to be taken into account when multiple media are to be adapted to computer devices can be derived from the facts mentioned above.

3.3. Computer-Based Media Standards

The first two of the natural human media (= information types) adapted to computers are well understood on the first glance. The handling of image and sound data has a long history in computer time-scales. So, there exist a number of standards.

Image:	Bitmap - TIFF, GIF, etc.
	Vector - HPGL, etc.
	Metafiles - CGM, Windows Metafiles, etc.
	Animated Images - Autodesk Animator, etc.
	Video - QuickTime, AVI, (MPEG), etc.

Sound: Noise - AIFF, U-LAW, WAVE, etc.
Speech - ADPCM, etc.
Music - MIDI, etc.

The tactile medium is of growing interest, especially if it comes to virtual-reality systems. But so far, there is no common file format to store and process tactile information.

For the discussions to follow, smell and taste are not taken into account, because they seem not to be needed for multimedia applications of the near future. Nevertheless, on the long run, they may become more important and basic research work should be done.

The major problem there will be I/O devices, file formats, and processing methods.

3.4. Quality and Reliability of Multimedia Services

As can be seen in chapter 3.2., the quality of graphical media needs to be sophisticated for the natural human capabilities are very high when it comes to "seeing."

Nowadays the different raster formats provide high resolution concerning number of colors and pixels. But when it comes to scalability and cross-platform interoperability they are still poor. On the other hand, losing single units of information (pixels) does not destroy the whole picture. So raster images are easy to use with respect to reliability. This is even more essential for moving raster images.

Vector formats provide a very good scalability. The resulting picture only depends on the capabilities of the output device. But only very few images can be stored vector-oriented besides CAD applications. Moreover, if only single information units (vectors) are lost, the whole image may be ruined.

Metafile formats combine raster and vector images, but cannot solve all problems concerning quality and reliability.

So, what would be necessary is a file format that allows the usage of raster data, is scalable, and is fault-tolerant. A first step may be the fractal analysis of raster images, what allows the reconstruction of the original image to an extend selectable by the user. Scalability is the major issue here. That means size, resolution, colors, etc. must be free parameters, only dependent of the original image, the processing power of the target system, and the user needs. Moreover, the data has to be so fault-tolerant that lost information units will not spoil the whole image. Existing raster image formats might be extended into this direction.

For sound formats the problem seems not to be so difficult. The "spatial" resolution is not as high as with images. Therefore, lost information is not so relevant. Moreover, very sophisticated algorithms concerning error detection in music and speech are in the market.

3.5. Interoperability

The interoperability comes into account when communication is concerned. The same media files are to presented or to be produced on different hardware and software platforms. So, common interchange formats have to be defined, focusing on network communication and storage in databases.

In order to achieve real-time communication, all involved machines need to exchange a set of set-up information in order to know about each others I/O, storage, processing, and interaction capabilities.

3.6. Intermixing Multimedia Data Types

The intermixing of multimedia data streams is mainly relevant for highly time-dependent media. All the others can be combined by simple relative synchronization methods like "start together," "stop together," "start B after A was running for x time units," "start B when A stops," etc.

Highly time-dependent media like animation sequences, videos, speech, etc. need more sophisticated methods, for playback as well as for real-time purposes. So the intermixing of animation, video, and audio files is very important. First steps have been taken with QuickTime and AVI, combining different media into one file format. In the development of adequate tools and applications based on these standardization efforts can be seen as a major issue of the future. This is especially needed for CSCW application, where fast communication and multimedia data exchange is essential.

4. Access Information: Computer Supported Cooperative Work

4.1. General Remarks About the Information Type "Access Information"

While there exist also stand-alone multimedia systems, it is often the case, that multimedia systems are used to support working groups. Therefore, consensus was reached that, when discussing the architecture of multimedia systems, also the problem of cooperative access has to be taken into account. It turned out, that the aspects of cooperative access can be seen orthogonal to the aspects of handling multiple media.

4.1.1. CSCW Based on Access Information. Computer-Supported Cooperative Work (CSCW) is seen to be based on an own information type, called access information. Therefore, the aspects of CSCW can be seen independent of the aspects of contents (media) and organization (hyper structures).

4.1.2. CSCW and Conferencing: Computer Conferencing. One aspect of CSCW is to provide a conferencing environment for the involved working group. Such conferencing environments are based on the following types of communications:

- point-to-point communication
- multipoint communication
- multicasting
- broadcasting

Conferencing may be supported by computers. Typical examples for this support are:

- shared screens
- multipointers
- telepointing

This then leads more and more to computer-supported conferencing, or computer conferencing.

4.1.3. CSCW and Computing: Conference Computing. Besides conferencing, CSCW also provides a computing environment. Computing environments may be distinguished according to the following characteristics:

- degree of freedom
- shared screen (follow user)
- individual screens
- social roles
- reader
- writer
- chairman
- interactivity
- static sessions
- dynamic sessions

With increasing conferencing capabilities, we approach the conference computing.

4.1.4. The Concept of a Cooperative Document: Private Annotations. One of the characteristics of computing in a conference is the concept of a cooperative document. In traditional systems, a document is represented by a file, having certain access rights. In a cooperative environment, a document (e.g., an electronic book) is shared by multiple users at the same time. Therefore, it is essential that users can make personal annotations to this document, and, herewith, privatize a copy.

4.1.5. Classification of CSCW Environments. CSCW environments may be distinguished between the following categories:

- same time/same place
- same time/different place
- different time/same place
- different time/different place

This has consequences for the implementation of the functions mentioned above as follows:

- communication:
  - same time: conferencing
  - different time: mailing
- computing:
  - same time: interactive conference computing
  - different time: cooperation of working groups

4.2. CSCW and Multimedia

A detailed look at multimedia is given in chapter 3. Here, we only add some comments concerning the usage of multimedia in CSCW environments. Multimedia has two impacts on CSCW: It may be used as a tool for communication as well as a contents of a cooperative document.

4.2.1. Multimedia as a Communication Tool. For CSCW at the same time (interactive CSCW), interactive communication between the users is essential. This means, that at least an efficient audio connection must be provided. Video can be seen as a meaningful add-on.

As mentioned earlier, different kinds of communication have to be implemented to support for example the different cooperation environments:

- point-to-point: for dialog environment
- hot-keys: to enable dialog communication in cooperative environments (passing the microphone)
- multicast: for building subgroups in large environments
- broadcast: for anonymous teleteaching.

4.2.2. Multimedia as Document Contents. When dealing with cooperative documents, we have to consider the facts that now different users may have access to different contents information and that the contents of such a document have to be presented to different screens at the same time.

4.2.3. Multimedia User Interfaces. In a cooperative environment, one has to deal with at least the following different information types:

- access information
- contents information
- structural information

The user interface has to reflect this fact. Effective presentation and interaction tools to deal with these information types have to be provided. It could be useful to associate different media with different information types. For example, requests from other users could be presented as sound even if they are not caused by spoken input.

4.3. CSCW and the View of Functional Categories

The concept of CSCW has an impact on all of the functional categories mentioned above.

4.3.1. CSCW and Processing. Concerning processing, algorithms for the following problems have to be developed:

- access management
- user identification
- user authorization
- ...

4.3.2. CSCW and Storage/Retrieval. Compared to the storage in a single user environment, the following additional issues arise:

- fine-grained transactions (very small access units)
- integration of (dynamic) access rights into the data base, reflecting the current status of the actual session

4.3.3. CSCW and Presentation/Interaction. Concerning the user interface, new metaphors have to be developed and implemented. The access status of a cooperative document has to be presented, allowing the user to see what parts of a document are free and which ones are used be others. When accessing an entity, conflicts may occur. Especially in large and widely distributed platforms, the update time and, herewith, the recognition of such problems may take a while. The user has to be informed about such situations (e.g., by a message "negotiating...").

An other important issue is to require document entities currently used by others. This can be done by conferencing, but also by sending a message and, for example, highlighting the requested zone.

Especially interesting is CSCW for hyper-documents. Tools have to be developed to get access to hierarchically structured information.

4.3.4. CSCW and Transfer/Communication. The concept of CSCW puts special requirements onto the transfer/communication functionality. As in other distributed multiuser applications, CSCW is based on the notion of a transaction. Requests have to be checked, a time stamp must be attached and access conflicts have to be detected and solved.

4.4. CSCW and Application Integration

CSCW, as mentioned earlier, is based on the information type "access information." Therefore, there is an intrinsic difference between cooperative and non-cooperative applications.

4.4.1. Generic Cooperation Support: Shared Applications. The idea of Generic Cooperation Support is to embed traditional applications in a cooperative environment. Here, the whole document underlying the application is seen as a single access entity. All users have the same rights, conceptually, we see a single user, but multiplicated application.

4.4.2. Joint Applications. In joint applications, still the document is a single access entity. However, the communication features are more elaborated. The write access right to the document may change during the session, and there may be a hierarchy of users. An example may be the blackboard in a classical teaching environment, where the teacher and the students may have write access, but the teacher has the privilege to give the access right. This type of application still can be implemented as a "conference computing shell" over a traditional application.

4.4.3. Cooperative Applications. In true cooperative applications, the access information is an inherent part of the underlying data structures. The underlying document now consists of several access entities (fine-grained access). Several users may have write access to different access entities in the same(!) document and at the same time.

5. Data Management

Multimedia systems have different requirements with respect to the management of their data. First, short-term storage must be distinguished from long-term storage. While the former deals with manipulations, direct access, specific formats, real-time, and synchronization, the latter has to cope with large data volumes, storage device management, heterogeneous environments (in space and time), search requests, and compression methods. Short-term storage is determined by the application and the computer system used, long-term storage must be much more general. Short-term storage can be further subdivided into main memory (not yet applicable to sound and video of reasonable size) and local secondary storage.

Second, the different media can be discussed. They have already been characterized in chapter 3, and these characteristics lead to many different requirements on data management. Some of the media are time-dependent, others are not. They all consist of a large number of small elements (e.g., characters or pixels), but these elements have very little in common and are arranged in different patterns, e.g., as set, sequence, or matrix.

Third, data management can be used to represent the organization of large numbers of media data objects. Hyperstructure is one example of such an organization, but not the only one. Media objects can also be organized in sets, either disjunct or overlapping. This can be used to classify them (e.g., X-rays, landsat photos, aerial photos).

Finally, the third dimension of the CHM cube is also relevant for data management: Access to the data can be supported in many different ways. They have to be located, either navigational or descriptive, and then interpreted. Concurrent access from several users should be allowed, but should be coordinated to preserve consistency. In particular, atomic sequences of updates on various data (transactions) should be supported.

5.1. What is a Multimedia Database?

A multimedia database is a large collection of media data objects on secondary (non-volatile) storage. Any such collection can be regarded as a data base. However, it makes a big difference how such a collection is managed. The operating system (OS) is in control of the external storage devices and offers low-level functionality to use them. It is suggested that there should be an additional data management system in between the application and the OS. However, long-term storage will need a different data management system than short-term storage.

A multimedia database management system (MMDBMS) enhances the functionality of a multimedia system with respect to the long-term storage and retrieval of multimedia data objects. The user may archive multimedia data objects and later search the archive. The objects are accessed not only by name (identifier), but also in a navigational and descriptive way.

Such an archive is also used to share data among a group of users. So data moved into the archive can be made available to others. Certain modes of information exchange and cooperation are supported by this.

Finally, the archive serves as a kind of public or corporate library. It offers access to standards, guidelines, templates, background info, legal info, etc.

It is important for the user not to be bothered with the specifics of matching his/her local facilities (workstation, peripherals) with those of the database server. Instead, the server should adapt to the environment of each particular user. So if the user wants to see an image, listen to a sound recording, or watch a video, he/she should be able to do so without selecting formats, converters, viewers, etc. In a first step, the system should offer a default viewing/listening mode (making the best of available resources). At wish, the user could then customize the presentation.

5.2. DB versus File Handling

Deciding about using either a DBMS or a file system is not so much an issue of end-user functionality but of system implementation. The same functionality (see 4.1) can be achieved with either a DBMS or a file system. There will be a difference in speed, in cost, and in maintenance effort. However, the implementation of some functionality (e.g., sharing and multiuser operation) requires a significant effort if done with a file system. Hence, in discussing the functionality of either the file system or the MMDBMS, we are talking about an API, not a UI (see 4.5).

File system and DBMS are two different "instances" of the service named "data/information structures." They offer different (internal) service to the application programmer.

The advantages of using a file system are:

- immediately available
- low cost
- highly optimized solutions possible (but not guaranteed)
- efficiency
- performance, speed (saving milliseconds)

The advantages of a (to be developed) MMDBMS are:

- independence of application programs (and toolkits) from storage and compression technology
- data abstraction (application neutrality, openness)
- explicit type info (metadata) for multimedia data objects
- "integration" with formatted data
- represent action of (typed) relationships
- powerful and efficient search facilities
- consistency (centralized control)

- multiuser operation with fine-grained concurrency control
- fault-tolerance (transactions, logging and recovery)
- potential for incremental and global optimization (single point of control)
- maintenance support after changes in environment (new clients, new storage technology; saving man-months)

It should also be noted that there are intermediate solutions. A system that offers data independence but not multiuser operation and transactions is much smaller than a full-fledged DBMS and thus also cheaper. Unfortunately, toady's commercially available DBMS cannot be tailored to that extent.

The choice should be made be the application programmer depending on the needs (and the budget) of the application.

In the following, we shall use the generic term "data management system" to refer to both a file system (plus application-specific functionality) and a DBMS.

5.3. Dynamic Data/Time Dependencies

DBMS until now had to cope with static data only. However, there has been some work on real-time databases, where queries had to be executed under tough timing constraints [SIGMOD88a]. The technology is there, but due to the limited market, only a few systems are commercially available on the specialized platforms used in real-time applications.

Here, it is very important that the data management system can distinguish types of data (and does not just offer containers for bytes). Storage management for time-based data should be guided by the real-time requirements. For instance, to achieve the required bandwidth in I/O, disk-striping can be used. Also, an appropriate storage device must be chosen.

So, only if the information about timing and time constraints is available to the data management system, it can react and provide specific means to obey them.

5.4. IIF versus Image Data Types

A format is a set of rules about how to code the media object. It defines a (physical) layout for the media object. Representation and coding are synonyms of format. A media object must have a format to exist, i.e., to be stored anywhere.

A type identifies a set of operations that allow to work with a (media) data object without knowing the format. The implementation of the operations can use different formats in different environments, still belonging to the same type. To design a proper set of operations is a difficult task.

The system should maintain and use metadata that provide information about the type (and format) of the data objects.

In short-term storage, usually very specific formats are used that match the local tools. There is no need to encapsulate them as types. The long-term archive however must cope with many different formats. To avoid redundancy, it will map them to the most general and/or most efficient format and encapsulate this. The create operator of the media data type thus accepts any format as input and converts it into the internal storage format used. The retrieve operator on the other hand can provide the client application with the format it needs. So, in the "create" and "retrieve" operations one has to identify the format used locally, and the data management system decides about the internal format to use.

While there are many formats, there is still a need for good types!

5.5. End-User Interface to Data Management

As said before, the data management system is considered to be of main use for the programmer of the multimedia application, not the end-user. Nevertheless, once the functionality of a DMS is fixed, it could also be made available to the end-user to let him/her look into the system and learn about the implementation (meaning?) of the higher-level functionality.

However, this should be compared to reading the output of a compiler, or even worse: to modifying it. The interface is designed to rather low-level. As a consequence, you can do more, but you have to do it in smaller steps.

5.6. Interoperability

Interoperability of DMS means the enhancement of a single DMS instance so that it can be accessed as one of several DMS instances (maybe at different sites) that cooperate to provide an answer to a query or to allow for consistent updates. The problems of schema integration, transaction management, and query optimization have not been solved for standard formatted data [Brei90a], so it seems to be too early to attack them with the additional burden of multimedia data objects. Some of the proposals for object-oriented database systems might extend to the management of multimedia data as well.

6. Communications

6.1. Requirements on Communication Services for Multimedia Applications

Due to the mass of data to be transferred in distributed multimedia systems, the overall requirements on communication services are very high speed and almost unlimited bandwidth. Exchange of data has to be executed in realtime and isochronously, i.e., the elapsed time required to transfer a certain amount of data must be predictable. The data transfer services should be fault-tolerant and reliable. Security aspects of data exchange in common networks have to be considered.

From the users or application programmers point of view all those aspects are summarized using the term "Quality of Services."

6.2. Standards

Obviously, standards for communication protocols are very important if data exchange in wide area or metropolitan area networks is considered. Unfortunately, the complexity of higher levels of protocol standards limits the peak performance provided by high-speed networks. On the other hand these protocols are more convenient for application programmers.

Most of toady's networks and standards for communication protocols do not fulfill the requirement of isochronity.

6.3. Trade-Offs in Communication Protocols

Mechanisms to provide fault-tolerance and security require additional data exchange and database queries. These are considered to be an overhead by programmers and users of applications which transfer huge volumes of data in short time.

6.4. Quality and Reliability of Services/Servers

Redundancies of servers, workers and services in a distributed system increase the fault-tolerance if any component in the entire system should be out of order.

6.5. Client/Server Architectures for Multimedia

In a client/server architecture the server and the communication channels of the server might be a bottleneck as far as high volume data transfer is concerned. It is more evident the more clients rely on a single server. On the other hand the distribution of common data over many nodes in the network requires additional services to ensure the consistency of the distributed databases at any time.

6.6. Interoperability

Interoperability is defined as the capability of autonomous systems to cooperate on a common task and solve a common problem.

7. Development Support

7.1. Implementers and Users

When talking about tools for multimedia we have to distinguish the implementer of multimedia functionality and the user of multimedia functionality, e.g., the author of a system with a multimedia user interface.

At the moment due to the variety of technical problems in the area of multimedia it is impossible to give an overview of the desired toolkits for multimedia implementers. So let us focus on tools and toolkits for authors of systems using multimedia.

Multimedia scene in nowadays reminds me of the early times of personal computing when you could make good money by building and selling your own word processor. Like word processors multimedia applications will become widely used and so, for being able to build many multimedia applications well fitted to the enduser's needs, we need standards, platforms and powerful toolkits.

7.2. Services

What we need for multimedia is something like X is for computer graphics. We need a (software) platform that reduces users deal with hardware dependencies to a minimum. Of course, the user still has to take into account what functionality he can get on a specific hardware platform. But it should not be his problem how to get it.

- These services should be hardware independent.
- The services should be offered to the user both on local and remote host in the same way.

- These services should include capture, presentation, transport across the network, storage and processing of multimedia objects.

7.3. Tools and Toolkits

We need a toolkit that allows the author to deal with multimedia objects—not with a lot of bits and bytes. This toolkit should provide a set of basic multimedia objects and should map the functionality of these basic objects onto the platform mentioned above.

Properties of this toolkit:

- Openness towards new interaction media
- Object-Orientation

Each object offers the author/user all properties changeable and all operations executable in the specific situation.

- Direct Composition

No programming needed for specifying layout of a user interface. Less programming needed for specifying the interactive behavior by use of spatialization of structure and time.

- Dynamic behavior can be defined interactively.
- Integration with graphical user interfaces.
- Use of MM in the Design-Process.

7.4. Application Framework

The construction of the application framework should be done by means of the toolkit, not by programming. To achieve this goal some requirements have to be made for the toolkit:

Aggregation. The toolkit allows the author to combine objects to a single more complex object. The author defines interactively the dynamic behavior of the whole object, the dynamic behavior of the parts of the object and the relations between them. In this way the author defines application specific object (or classes).

Example: Medical Doctors often want to mark an "area of interest" in X-ray images. The author combines a container element, a pixmap and a polyline to a new object of the kind of "X-ray image." The author defines: The polyline is invisible. When the user (the medical doctor) clicks on the image, a visible copy of the polyline is created and the polyline changes according to users mouse movements. In this way no programming was necessary to create a application specific object. Each object contains its design functionality.

8. Conclusions

The goal of this working group was to identify views on multimedia architectures. To reach this goal, first different aspects of multimedia systems have been identified and isolated. This has led to a more detailed investigation of media as the basic contents information and computer-supported cooperative work based on access information. Requirements of multimedia user interfaces in cooperative environments have been stated. Data management and communication as central components have also be investigated. At the end, the working group has discussed aspects of development support for multimedia applications.

Altogether, this report reflects the different options stated in the two days working group discussions and may serve as a first initial step towards the development of a reference model for multimedia system architectures.

9. References

[Brei90a] Breitbart, Y., "Multidatabase Interoperability," ACM SIGMOD Record, vol. 19, no. 3, Sept. 1990, pp. 53-60.

[SIGMOD88a] ACM SIGMOD Record, Special Issue on Real-Time Database Systems, vol. 17, no. 1, March 1988.

[Stei90a] Steinmetz, R., Rückert, J., und Racke, W., "Multimedia-Systeme," Das aktuelle Schlagwort, Informatik-Spektrum, Bd. 13, H. 5, S. 280-282 (in German).

Group III Report: Digital Video in Multimedia Systems

Group III Members: Bernd Girod, Ralf Guido Herrtwich, Georg Rainer Hofmann, Takahiko Kamae, Meinrad Niemöller, Stefan Noll, Ralf Steinmetz, Ana Sofia Vieira

1. Introduction

The integration of motion video into computer systems offers many new opportunities for multimedia applications. Unfortunately, it also implies a variety of technical problems still to be overcome. The data rate of a raw video signal in PCM format can be more than 100 Mbit/s. On the other hand, the bandwidth available on computer busses, mass storage devices, and local area networks is typically a lot smaller. For example, Ethernet has a peak rate of 10 Mbit/s, typical hard disks will support a sustained rate up to 10 Mbit/s, a CD-ROM runs at a few Mbit/s, ISDN has a rate of 64 kbit/s. Thus, data compression is a key technology to integrate motion video into computers.

Video compression has made great progress in the last ten years, however, it has been developed and optimized for broadcasting and videotelephony applications. With a few exceptions, these developments have assumed a fixed rate digital channel with negligible error rate and well-defined parameters of the video source and the display. Only recently, there has been an increasing awareness of the special requirements that have to be met for the integration of digital video into computer systems.

This report summarizes the results of discussions of a working group (Working Group III) that was formed during the 1992 Dagstuhl workshop on "Multimedia System Architectures and Applications," being held from November 2nd to 4th in 1992. We have focused on fully digital integration of motion video into the computer. Currently, there are many systems that combine motion video and computers by controlling analog video devices. We are not discussing these systems here, since they will probably disappear as soon as there are fully integrated digital solutions. In our work, we concentrated on open system architectures that are typical for a workstation or personal computer environment. We are aware, however, that there are many multimedia applications for the consumer market, where closed systems (such as CD-I) are likely to prevail. Many of our conclusions hold for both types of systems.

This report is structured as follows. In Section 2, we outline a few typical application scenarios and attempt a classification of applications. In Section 3, we summarize the requirements that result for video compression schemes for the different classes of applications. Section 4 discusses the performance and features of some of the proposed compression methods, both standardized and proprietary. Scalable video is such an important topic that we devoted the entire Section 5 to it, while Section 6 discusses issues arising from the relationship between video and other media modalities, such as the representation of still images or synchronization with audio.

2. Video Applications

In the area of multimedia systems, there is a considerable number of applications which make intensively use of information types which are referred to by terms as

(1) analogous and digital video,
(2) motion pictures,
(3) image sequences,
(4) time-variant images,
(5) and the like.

The variety of the above listed terms shows that it is worth to consider

(6) the underlying structures,
(7) the kind of user interaction, and
(8) the corresponding data types

which are employed by the various applications. The following paragraphs illuminate these applications.

2.1. Application Scenarios

The following paragraphs describe—exemplary versus exhaustive—some applications in more detail.

Aspen Video Map. The Aspen Video Map has been one of the early developments in the area of interactive video systems (at MIT, in the late 1970s). It is a collection of realworld video sequences which have been taken from the city of Aspen, Colorado. The video sequences show in essence drive-through pictures from the various streets and places of the city. These video sequences are arranged as "clips" in a storage-and-retrieval system. On a map, the user may interactively select the street or place he would like to see. The system retrieves and displays the according video sequence.

Karaoke. In the area of consumer-electronics-oriented multimedia systems which are serving for entertainment, for leisure, or as electronic games, Karaoke is of increasing importance for the Japanese market. Karaoke systems are presentation-only systems for the multimedia presentation of "songs" for singing-along. A video/audio sequence is displayed simultaneously with the text of the song—whereas the audio is containing only the background music. The actual parts—which correspond to the background music—of the text are highlighted.

Video-On-demand (on-line/off-line). Systems for video-on-demand are oriented towards the consumer and home video market. The basic idea is that the user—in contrast to the traditional television system—shall not be restricted to the watching of centrally broadcasted TV programs. Instead, the user may interactively select from a list—comparable to videotext tables—of films, shows, etc., what he would like to see. The selected TV program is then sent to the user's home TV set either in the "on-line" or the "off-line" modus. In case on-line modus is used, the selected TV program is distributed from a central TV program supplier via broadband networks to the user. The user's system is a presentation-only system, with no need to store the distributed TV program. For the off-line modus, the selected TV program is send to the user not necessarily in realtime. Therefore, for distribution, narrowband networks may be employed, as well as network-independent data storage devices (like laser discs, etc.). In case a network is employed, the user's TV-like device must intermediately store the distributed TV program, until the user would like to watch it.

Videophony. Videophony—sometimes referred to as "picture telephone" as well—is a point-to-point (with 2 participants), or even multipoint (more than 2 participants, see also CSCW below), telecommunication service. Videophony allows for the signal-oriented transmission of both, video and audio. According to the bandwidth of the network, however, the image quality of the transmitted video may be reasonable low, both in terms of spatial and temporal resolution of the video. To meet this problem, the videophony standards (such as CCITT Rec H.261) make intensive use of sophisticated compression algorithms, which include transform coding, motion prediction and compensation, and the like.

TV/Video on LAN. Some videophony-like applications use local area networks (LANs) for the inhouse (local) communication of TV/Video signals and/or the according data streams. Those applications may include the "netcasting" of audio and/or video messages, e.g., inhouse announcements and/or bulletins. Other applications may be surveillance-oriented, where video data is transmitted —either occasionally or permanently—over LANs for the centralized monitoring of facilities. This may include also user interaction to allow, e.g., for the remote steering of camera positions, and the like.

CSCW/Multipoint Conferencing. There is a number of applications for collaborative work. These are affecting technical, e.g., CAD-oriented, work as well as meeting and workshop scenarios. For workshop and meeting scenarios, the following points have to be taken into consideration:

- Multipoint interconnection needs to be established. Typical numbers of conference participants range from at least 2 up to 4 to 5. Groups with more than 6 conferencing participants are becoming increasingly un suitable for teleconferencing.
- A "forum" situation must be achieved, where passing over and taking the conference chair, the floor (for speaking up), and stepping into a dis cussion needs to be provided by the system
- The privacy of the user must be shielded against unwelcome visual insights. That is, the user must not be watched by cameras in his office/ private space unless he explicitly wants it.
- The spontaneous setting-up of conferencing sessions (especially for point-to-point connections) must be achievable. The corresponding confer encing hardware systems and telecommunication terminals—under ideal conditions—shall be implemented as desktop systems.
- For conferencing not only video and audio is needed, but communication needs also to be assisted by telematic services, such as:
  - transmission of high-resolution still images, to allow for the readability of text with even smaller letters,
  - for point-to-point connections: telewriting, which provides vector-graphics shared sketchpad functionality incl. hardcopy,
  - for multipoint connections: shared whiteboard, whose functionality maybe quite comparable to the telewriting devices.
- The conferencing equipment must be affordable in terms of financial investments per workstation and/or per user.

Multimedia Mail. Multimedia Mail forms extensions to the well-known email systems, as provided by, e.g., the message handling systems (MHS) specified by CCITT Rec X.400 series. This is achieved by extending the functionality of the "messages" which can be handled and passed forward by the MHS. Therefore, the message structure's capability is increased by adding the "multimedia" data types (still image, image sequence, audio, etc.) as additional message body part types. The traditional modus of store-and-forwarding mail messages, as used by the MHS, is applied to the Multimedia Mail systems and applications.

2.2. Classification of Scenarios

Taking into account the above mentioned scenarios, a classification of these, with respect of the functionality of user interaction, can be given and characterized as follows:

(A) Broadcasting. The user may select among the broadcasted channels and programs the one that he would like to watch on his receiver set. The user may step in and out the broadcasted program by switching ON/OFF the receiver device.

(B) Interactive Retrieval. The user may select among the provided pieces of multimedia information, which is, e.g., select by title or by index. The system provides typically capabilities for the playing/displaying the information, as well as searching, fastforwarding, and rewinding through the multimedia documents. In contrast to broadcasting, the user may additionally halt/pause the information retrieval, and resume later on. Of course, It is also possible, in contrast to broadcasting, to retrieve the document's information repeatedly.

(C) Editing. The editing of document necessarily encompasses the functionality of the interactive retrieval of documents (see paragraphs above). Referring to the retrieval as a "read" functionality, editing must encompass also a "write" functionality as well, in order to allow for the storage of multimedia information. For editing, two areas need to be distinguished carefully:

- The editing of data structures (as described by syntactical rules).
- The editing of contents (as described by semantical contexts).

(D) Conferencing. The functionality which needs to be provided to the user by conferencing systems may be grouped as follows:

- Broadcasting functionality; see chapter (A) above. There may be participants allowed to attend at—even one or more—conferences who have an "observer" status. For these, it is essential to step in/out the ongoing conferences.
- Information retrieval functionality; see chapter (B) above.
- Editing functionality; see chapter (C) above.
- Floor control functionality: The floor, which includes to handle and pass over the right to speak up, as well to step into the ongoing debate, must be controlled by the chair. By separate mechanisms, the role of the chair may be passed over to another participant.

- Workspace and device management: The use and the # of the available telematic services (telewriting, shared whiteboard, etc.) must be controlled by the conference.

3. Criteria for Video Compression Schemes

The sheer amount of digital video (which is 216 Mbit/s for CCIR 601 encoded television images) leads to the need for compressing it when the data is stored or exchanged with today's computing equipment. To arrive at a data volume that this equipment is able to handle, compression by a factor of at least 100 is required. Using today's technology, this is only achievable with lossy compression.

A general problem for every lossy compression algorithm is to reduce the amount of data to the maximum extent possible while still providing acceptable (or appropriate) video quality, low algorithmic complexity, and short compression delay. Whereas rate, complexity, and delay can be measured easily, video quality can hardly be determined in an objective manner. To determine whether a compression algorithm yields the desired level of quality, one usually chooses a set of video sequences typical for a particular application domain and empirically lets a larger number of users evaluate the compressed samples. In general, the application domains in Section 2.2 require the following levels of quality:

Applic. Scenario:	**Level of Quality:**	**Example:**
Broadcasting:	medium high	(TV "broadcast quality")
Interactive Retrieval:	medium low	(VHS quality)
Editing:	high	(television studio quality)
Conferencing:	low	(below VHS quality)

How much data a compression algorithm produces or generates within a certain amount of time determines the bit rate of the data stream. Yet, the mere information of bit/s provides no information about the sophistication of a compression method as it is not related to the underlying raw data, e.g., the image size. How good a compression algorithm is can better be characterized by the compression ratio achieved; it can be measured in bit/pixel. Good compression algorithms for motion video today achieve a compression ratio below 1 bit/pixel. With this compression ratio, the following bit rates have turned out to provide the appropriate quality for the above mentioned applications (thereby also providing a more precise quality measurement):

Application Scenario:	**Bit Rate:**
Broadcasting:	5-10 Mbit/s
Interactive Retrieval:	1-5 Mbit/s
Editing:	5-20 Mbit/s
Conferencing:	0.05-2 Mbit/s

How complex a compression algorithm is depends on its processing and memory requirements. Algorithmic complexity determines above all whether the compression can take place in real time, i.e., whether before the arrival of the next video frame all compression steps for the previous frame have been computationally completed. Arguably, one can also measure complexity in terms of hardware required to perform the compression task—both in terms of speed and in terms of cost. For our applications, complexity requirements are as follows:

(1) Broadcasting: Can be high for compression, should be low or medium for decompression.

(2) Interactive Retrieval: Can be high for compression, should be low or medium for decompression.

(3) Editing: Should be low.

(4) Conferencing: Should be low.

The delay of a compression algorithm, i.e., the time it takes for the algorithm to process a frame, obviously also determines its interactive qualities. Application requirements on end-to-end or roundtrip delay impose restrictions on the time the compression may take. For the applications we consider, the requirements on delay reflect the tolerance on complexity:

Application Scenario:	**Bit Rate:**
Broadcasting:	below 1 s
Interactive Retrieval:	well below 1 s
Editing:	below 150 ms
Conferencing:	below 150 ms

Apart from these major criteria for evaluating the appropriateness of a certain compression technique, several additional features of a video compression scheme should be considered. These include:

(1) Random access: Certain applications do not access a video stream sequentially from the start, but start playing it from an arbitrary position; they may browse through the stream in fast forward or rewind mode or even play the stream backwards. For these applications, random access to all positions within the stream is required. For interactive retrieval and

editing applications, random access is a must. It is usually not required for broadcasting and conferencing.

(2) Editability: Not all compression formats lend themselves easily to editing the video data. In general, the extent to which interframe encoding is used determines the ease of editing: The more individual images stand for themselves, the easier the editing process is. Obviously, editability and random access are tightly coupled.

(3) Symmetry: A compression algorithm is called symmetric if compression and decompression take about the same number of operations. Today, symmetric algorithms are used for realtime interaction, whereas asymmetric algorithms are applied to one-way communication. Symmetric is, hence, desired for editing and conferencing, whereas asymmetric algorithms can be found in the broadcasting and information retrieval domains.

(4) Robustness: How robust a decompression algorithm is depends on its ability to cope with bit or message errors in the video stream to be processed. In distributed environments the exchange of video streams across a network may induce such errors. Neither should these errors cause the decompression algorithm to stop, nor should the errors become notable to the users. While robustness is a general requirement for all compression algorithms used in a distributed environment, it is a must in conferencing applications as these are always run across networks.

An additional requirement for video compression algorithm that results from the dynamic environment in which they are used is scalability. We delay the discussion of scalability to Section 5 and first examine how today's compression schemes meet the requirements outlined above.

4. Scalable Video

4.1. Definition of Scalable Video

In the discussion on the requirements of the different classes of video application scenarios we found that the scalability of video is highly desirable for all classes.

We define loosely scalable video as the ability of a system to adapt to a certain bandwidth "on the fly." Bandwidth of a system may be reduced by the allocation of computing or network resources to other tasks. In the dynamic environment of a multitasking system, it is therefore necessary to adaptively scale down or scale up the bandwidth of the video task.

To understand the usefulness of scalable video, it is helpful to consider human perception of visual information. It is a well-known fact that the image perceived by a human is progressively build up from a coarse resolution to finer detail. Moreover, the human perception process dynamically scales up the resolution around the focus of interest (point of view). We believe that computer scientists can learn a lot from the experiences made by television engineers when defining a coding scheme for TV broadcasting. This applies to the coding of still images as well as to the coding of motion video.

Experiments have shown that the relation between the bandwidth in terms of bits per second to the image quality perceived by humans is not linear. With increasing data rate the image quality quickly rises up, but then further increase of the data rate leads only to a slow, asymptotical increase of image quality towards a threshold.

4.2. Domains of Scaling

We do not understand scaling video as the mere change of the video image size. The scaling of the bandwidth of a video can be achieved in different domains:

Time: This is the most common approach; here, the rate of frames presented per second is changed dynamically. As we can see in TV technology a rate of 20 to 30 frames per second gives humans the impression of smooth movement. In case of, e.g., congestions on a network even a lower frame rate can be accepted.

Space: The resolution of a (video) image is defined by the number of pixels per viewing angle. An image can be progressively build up by increasing the number of pixels in a hierarchical fashion.

Frequency: If a image is transformed into the frequency domain, the bandwidth can be reduced by cutting the higher DCT-coefficients. The back-transformation then leads to unsharp images (loss of detail).

Amplitude: An image quantized with a resolution of 8 bits per pixel, e.g., can be reduced in bandwidth by cutting the least significant bits.

Color space: A resolution of 8 bits per color (red, green, blue) and pixel is called "true color" (24 bit). This brute force approach does not take the human perception into account. The TV coding with the its separation and subsampling of the chrominance and luminance signals is one approach to reduce overall bandwidth. Best results can be achieved by combinations of these approaches.

To review the different standards and proprietary schemes for compression of video in the context of scalability it is useful to identify some criteria:

Graceful degradation: In case of the drop of one or more frames the quality of the video image should not go down to zero but rather decrease in a graceful way. In this context it is also an important question how long a certain compression scheme needs to recover (e.g., from drops of frames) to full image quality.

Partial decoding: For the transmission of video over networks it is useful to progressively transmit the video images. For that, a compression scheme should allow for the partial decoding of the incoming chunks of video information.

4.3. Review of Standards

Based on these criteria and the characteristics outlined in chapter 4, we can review the standards and proprietary schemes:

MPEG-1: The MPEG-1 compression scheme is not scalable. We believe that the relevance of MPEG-1 could only arise from the mass production of dedicated chips, which will be not scalable. Because of the complex structure of I-, P-, and B-frames in MPEG-1 it is especially difficult to recover from frame drops (caused by network congestions).

MPEG-2: The follow-up of MPEG-1 will be scalable in the extent that the bandwidth will be allowed to drop from the MPEG-2 rates (5-20 Mbits/s) to MPEG-1 rate (1.5 Mbit/s).

JPEG and Motion-JPEG: Because there is no interframe compression in JPEG, is very easy to drop frames and also to recover from these drops.

px64 and H.26x: The px64- and H.26x-compression schemes are not scalable. Only future versions of the H.26x standards will address to the scalability problem.

Roadpizza: QuickTime's compression scheme Roadpizza makes use of scaling of bandwidth in the time domain (at least). The bandwidth can be dynamically adapted to the workload of the processor. Details are not known by the authors because of the proprietary character of the compression scheme.

Fluentlinks: Fluentlinks allows video communication across networks and uses a Motion-JPEG scheme with some proprietary add-ons.

4.4. Software-Codecs and Hardware-Bottlenecks

The scalability feature of a compression/decompression scheme is especially interesting when it comes to software-only realizations on general-purpose processors. Beside demanding workload-dependent scaling for decompression, software-codecs call also for simple and fast algorithms. The MPEG-1 standard is therefore not a good candidate for software-only realizations.

We expect that customers will more likely accept poor image quality with a cheap software-only solution today when they can expect better image quality with the next generation of general-purpose CPUs. In contrast to that, a customer subscribing to a hardware solution of a codec, e.g., a dedicated board, can only grade up to the next generation (of image quality) by throwing away the boards or plugging in new processors.

So, an interesting question is, when the different compression schemes can realized software-only on general-purpose CPUs. Projecting the last years progress of increase of CPU power into the future, we can expect to see software-only realizations of the MPEG-1 standard in about 4 to 5 years.

It is an open question how the development of other components of a general-purpose computer like RAM, bus and network adapter can keep pace with the development of CPUs. For the storing of video images not only a huge memory size is necessary, but also the access-time needs to be low. For the cooperation of (multiple) CPUs with the RAM the system bus needs to provide a high bandwidth.

5. Video Standards

5.1. Outline of Video Standards

Video standards consist mainly of a video format, a compression algorithm, and a data frame structure. There are two major kinds of analog TV system today:

- the 525/60 system (NTSC), and
- the 625/50 system (PAL, SECAM).

These two systems also form the basis for digital systems. To fill the gap of this two different system, a common video format is important, the so-called Common Intermediate Format (CIF). The Common Intermediate Format or CIF is the only existing video format that is globally recognized. The quarter CIF (QCIF) is the corresponding standardized low resolution format.

CIF is suitable for the usage at a bitrate 384 Kb/sec, or higher; while QCIF is suitable at a bitrate 64 Kb/sec or 128 Kb/sec.

Compression algorithms that currently applied in video standards are

- discrete cosine transform (DCT),
- motion compensation (MC),
- Interframe Interpolation, and
- variable length coding (VLC).

More efficient compression algorithms generally cause more coding delay. Reasonably low delay is required in the realtime video applications such video telephone and video conferencing. On the other hand, the requirement for coding delay is much less severe in the video storage applications such as video in compact disk or laser disk. Bi-directional interframe interpolation contributes greatly to high compression rate, although it increases coding by an order of several 100 msec. Data frame structure is necessary to find the start point and the break point of video data. In video telephone/conferencing, the frame structure also specifies a way to multiplex video, audio and control data.

5.2. International Video Standards

(1) MPEG-1 and H.261 JTC1 of ISO/IEC and CCITT SG15 cooperated to set the motion video standards called MPEG-1 and H.261. These video standards can be applied to a digital video at a bitrate of 2 Mb/sec, or lower. The main purpose of MPEG-1 is the video storage in the compact disk. The bi-directional interframe interpolation makes MPEG-1 more efficient than H.261. H.261, in turn, is suitable for video telephone and video conferencing. Both, MPEG-1 and H.261 are based on CIF.

(2) JPEG is the standard for full color still image. JPEG has been developed by JTC 1 of ISO/IEC. JPEG can be applied very widely from very fine color photographs to freeze frame video. Lossless coding of full color images can be done using JPEG. In the computer applications of motion video, JPEG is attractive because every frame of motion video can be independently encoded, and also decoding can start at any frame. In this kind of application, JPEG is frequently called Motion-JPEG or MJPEG.

(3) For MPEG-2 and H.26X, JTC 1 of ISO/IEC and CCITT SG15 are continuing their cooperation to set video standard for high quality motion video. The targeted quality is equivalent to, or even higher, than broadcast video quality. The necessary bitrate is generally believed to be somewhere between 5 and 10 Mb/sec. Scalable motion video is one of the most important features The standard is tentatively called MPEG-2 at the JTC-1 side and H.26X at the CCITT side; however they are believed to be defined identically.

5.3. Industry Video Standards

Several industry motion video standards are in use in multimedia workstations and packaged motion video.

(1) DVI (Digital Video Interactive) is INTEL's proprietary scheme. Encoding needs relatively high processing power, because DVI is mainly used for packed video. Thus, the encoding is done off-line using super computers. While DVI took a pioneering role, it will not be supported in the future.

(2) Apple Computers have introduced the proprietary Roadpizza compression scheme as part of their QuickTime software. Roadpizza is a fully scalable, highly asymmetric software codec, that supports the continuous image resizing and partial decoding of the bitstream. Image quality is still very low on the existing platforms, but it is getting better as new, more powerful computer are introduced.

(3) Fluent Inc. has developed a scalable compression scheme based on MJPEG that is intended for network applications. In the early product the receiving side monitors whether it receives frames too late and provides a massage back to the sender to reduce the frame rate to be sent.

5.4. Future Role of Video Standards

Video standards enable various binds of interworking. In realtime video applications, such as video telephone and video conferencing, terminals based on the international video standards can be interconnected at an international scale. The package media such as compact disc (CD) can be restored by any CD player in such a way that audio CD can be played in any part of the world. In the computer applications, standard video data can be interchanged through LAN and/or wide area networks. However, in the computer applications, software-only coding and decoding are frequently discussed. As computers become more powerful, software-only coding and/or decoding attracts more attention.

The role of video standards might change. Suppose that coding and decoding process can be written using a standard software language, video decoding software may be able to be transmitted prior to transmitting video data. Then any video data can be decoded. In such a situation, standardized video compression algorithms may not be necessary; scalable video formats standard may become more important.

6. Video and Its Relationship to Other Media

6.1. Synchronization with Audio

The main interdependence between video and audio results from the fact that typical videos have a soundtrack accompanying them. The synchronization of video with audio can be achieved in different ways. Depending on the granularity of synchronization there are two possibilities:

(1) start/stop synchronization,
(2) frame synchronization.

The start/stop synchronization defines a maximum tolerance between the start (and stop) of two media S1 and S2. The starts of the two media are synchronized by a trigger T1, which will be generated after the start of S1 and triggers the start of S2. The frame synchronization generates triggers for each frame. The triggers Ti can refer to

(a) relative next frame,
(b) absolute frame number,
(c) global time (GMT, CET, etc.).

In cases (a) and (b) the application uses an internal unique time. In case (c) the application refers to a global time system and an adjusting of the internal times (clocks) of each workstation/partner side is necessary. This could be done by handshaking to figure out the delay between source and sink, and sending of time stamps. Independent of the way of synchronization the interleaving of the audio and video data streams is useful to realize the synchronization.

For some multimedia applications in the domain of presenting documents the start/stop synchronization is sufficient, because of lower requirements. For example, in most MM applications video and audio come from the same source and the delay between the starts of audio and video will be small ($d < 150$ msec.). In conference applications there should be a global time synchronization and the requirement is to try to synchronize as closely as possible. For lip synchronization a frame synchronization is necessary.

6.2. Still Images / Documents

One video frame could be understood as one still image, and a still image could be understood as an image sequence of length 1 (one frame). The mathematical model for video images and still images is the same, except for the time parameter. This implies that image editing is the same as video content editing. But there are big differences in usage, applications, quality and compression. One example are the different viewing distances, when perceiving a video or a still image. Usually is a distance of 1 x diagonal length for still images and 4-6 times the diagonal length for video (i.e., contours are sharper viewable on motion pictures).

This will have an impact on user interfaces for workstation integrated video. In this context the distinction of still images into two classes is important:

(1) scanned images/photographic material,
(2) binary documents/object-oriented graphics.

Documents typically have a higher resolution than photographic material and video. For photographic material and video there can be used lossy compression algorithms. For video MPEG or M-JPEG was recommended, for photographics JPEG is useful (see above). For documents a lossless compression is needed. Possible standards are JBIG, G3/G4 FAX and TIFF. It was mentioned, that for some applications lossy compression is reasonable, but for legal reasons lossless compression is required (i.e., X-ray pictures). Scalability is important also for archiving still images (photographics).

7. Conclusions

In this report, we have summarized the results of discussions of a working group on "Video Integration" at the 1992 Dagstuhl Workshop on Multimedia System Architectures and Applications. Starting from a few prototypical applications, we have grouped applications into four classes. These application scenarios are

(1) broadcast-type,
(2) interactive retrieval,
(3) editing, and
(4) conferencing.

We have identified typical requirements with respect to image quality, delay, and information access. It turns out that scalability of the video representation is highly desirable for all application classes. This requirement arises from both the wish to resize video windows on the computer screen and the varying bandwidth limitations in computer systems. Software-only codecs will become feasible in the future, providing another strong motivation for scalability. We concluded that scalability needs to be supported from the maximum bandwidth down to zero.

Unfortunately, existing motion video compression standards such as CCITT H.261 or ISO MPEG-1 do not support scalability. Therefore, manufacturers are introducing their own proprietary schemes. M-JPEG, the extension of the intraframe coding scheme JPEG to video, has several desirable features, its compression ratio, however, is clearly inferior to interframe schemes. Future programmable platforms will probably support multiple compression algorithms. While CPUs powerful enough for realtime compression/decompression are expected within 5 years, it is not clear whether other bottlenecks in the computer architecture might possibly delay high-quality software-only codecs further.

For the integration of motion video into computers, we have to keep in mind its relationship to other media. Video is usually accompanied by audio, and provisions are required to synchronize these data streams. Still images and binary documents are media forms closely related to motion video. While there is a continuum between a fast slide show of still images and a low frame rate movie, still and moving images have typically very different requirements such that a separate treatment is the likely solution for the near future. Spatial scalability is important both for moving images and for still images.

In summary, there are several open research questions. The current compression standards for motion video are not satisfactory for computer applications. Most of the research questions are centered around the issue of scalable video. Scalable video is the key to fully integrate motion video into computers.

Second Section

Co-operative Multimedia on Heterogeneous Platforms

B. Tritsch and Ch. Hornung
Fraunhofer Institute for Computer Graphics, Wilhelminenstrasse 7, 64283 Darmstadt, Germany

Abstract

The development of a distributed and heterogeneous generic multimedia platform presents many issues. The hardware, software and network platforms are heterogeneous, so *device-independence* and *interoperability* are vital. Therefore, the primary objective of the research presented here is to introduce, to specify and to evaluate a generic architecture, including communication mechanisms and multimedia features. This architecture provides functionality in the areas of transfer, processing, storage, presentation and interaction. In addition, co-operation and timing control paradigms must be introduced to allow real-time communication and remote access; such features are termed *Tele-Media* (tele-communicating multimedia).

The implementation part of this paper highlights the real-time Tele-Media features of the generic architecture. First results show that such multimedia communication is possible with acceptable performance and at reasonable costs on standard platforms and networks.

1 Introduction

Multimedia is defined as the combination of three or more of text, graphics, animation, music, speech, images and video. The increasing use of multimedia brings with it a dramatic change in today's computer usage. The hitherto strong distinction between business and entertainment computer applications is becoming blurred due to the increasing integration of communication media (such as fax, radio and television), and fast, convenient access to multimedia information systems.

The eventual outcome of this increased communication must be the use of multimedia in all facets of life -- both in the office and at home. As part of this process, increased communication via network connectivity will see a move towards distance *co-operation* both in terms of computer conferencing and the multi-author preparation of *multimedia documents*.

1.1 Co-operative HyperMedia

The structure of multimedia documents might be very complex. Today, documents are mostly linearly structured (such as in most text processing systems) or hierarchically structured (such as graphics), but there is an increasing trend towards intelligent links. These links may be time-variant and may be associated with semantic functions. Such documents are termed *hyper-documents*.

In order to reach a higher level of abstraction, the term *Co-operative HyperMedia* (CHM) is introduced for documents (information units) and systems (information processing units).

A CHM system handles the processing, storage, transfer, presentation and interaction between CHM documents [1]. The different components of such a CHM document are:

- multimedia contents
- hyper structure organisation
- co-operative access

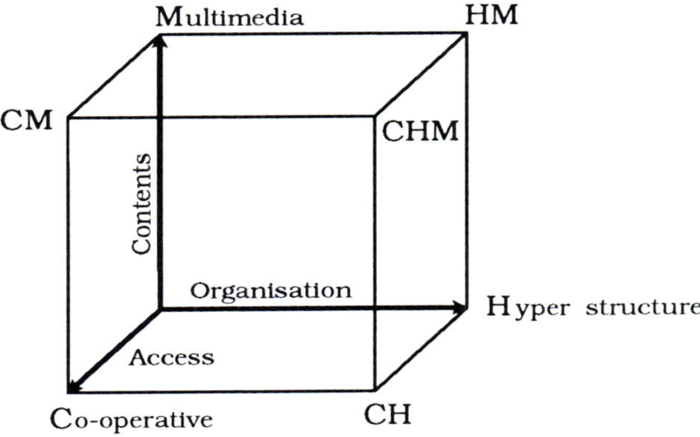

Fig. 1.1. The CHM cube

These three element types are orthogonal and can be represented by the axes of a three-dimensional object, the *CHM cube* (see figure 1.1). Time, as an additional element type, is incorporated into each of the three other element types.

1.2 Tele-Media

If this CHM model does indeed hold, the information and communication technologies should, eventually, join.

The main goal of today's computer communication is to be as close as possible to real human communication, where media such as voice, image and gesture should be accurately supported by the available computer technology. People and computers are placed in a time and space continuum. Two or more people may coincide in one or other of these dimensions, in both, or in neither [2]. During a live conversation, time and place are the same for two or more communicating partners. If one of the conversation partners stores and then forwards his message, then for the other partners the time is later, place may be different and hence the "live" or "real-time" characteristics of the conversation are lost. Today's information and communication technology allows partners to approximate the benefits of real-time interaction even when physical proximity is not feasible.

In distributed, co-operative multimedia systems, we need different exchangeable computer-based media, some with real-time capabilities. Here, we want to introduce *Tele-communicating Multimedia (Tele-Media)* mechanisms as we use them in our system, focusing on their timing and real-time features [1, 3].

Informally, a *Tele-Medium* is described as an information and communication channel based on multimedia input/output devices and electronic communication devices with a defined alphabet (protocol). Therefore, a Tele-Medium supports the on-line or off-line exchange of messages using this alphabet.

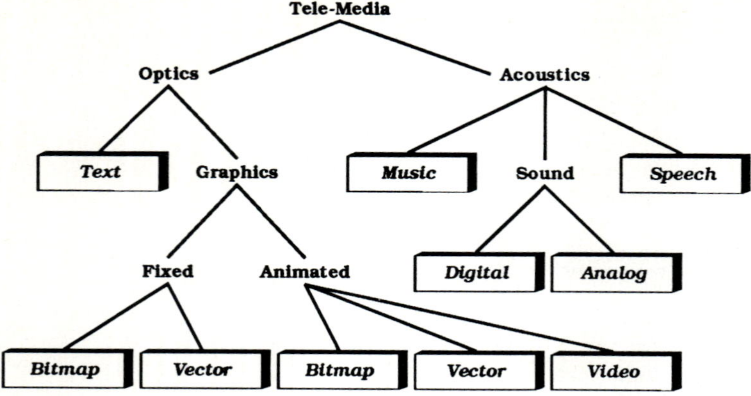

Fig. 1.2. The Tele-Media

According to their internal time-dependence, we distinguish between the following types of Tele-Media:

- *Static Tele-Media*, such as text and still images.
- *Dynamic Tele-Media*, such as animation, video and sound recorded and/or played back locally
- *Real-time Tele-Media*, such as real-time video and real-time sound

For static and dynamic Tele-Media, the information is typically one way -- experts author the material and users play it back. Prepared multimedia material may be retrieved or played back from sources such as CD-ROMs, on-line files, or the network. Real-time Tele-Media take this one step further, enabling real-time, asynchronous and interactive communication among a group of users. Here, the communication is two-way.

The primary goal of each Tele-Medium is to guarantee that the Medium is transmitted, received and played back correctly in time. This is referred to as *isochronity*. Moreover, the timing problems between two or more related dynamic or real-time multimedia objects have to be handled by the Tele-Media mechanisms. This is referred to as *synchronity*. Both isochronity and synchronity are based on precise time processing, to the resolution of milliseconds [4].

The Tele-Media mechanisms also incorporate more sophisticated features:

- *Remote control*, allowing execution, manipulation and synchronisation of Tele-Media over long distances
- Exception handling, taking care of possible data loss or delays
- *Cross-platform performance adaptation*, enabling co-operation between platforms with different performances
- *Multicast/multipoint communication*, allowing more than two users to communicate simultaneously
- *Compression/decompression*, reducing the Tele-Media data flow on the network

1.3 Multimedia Hardware Platforms

At least two networked multimedia workstations are prerequisite for co-operative multimedia. Connectivity, interoperability, speed, multi-tasking, multimedia capability, and client/server architectures are the key issues of future Workstation environments and should be achieved by applying commonly accepted standards and architectures.

Taking all these requirements into account, we decided to use the following standard hardware platforms as our heterogeneous development and evaluation environment: Sun Sparc 2/10, Silicon Graphics Indigo and Multimedia PCs. In addition, all workstations had to meet extended hardware requirements available either as part of the standard configuration or at reasonable cost (totally less than 50% of the standard Workstation price). The reason was that we wanted to address a broad group using networked workstations. The extended requirements mentioned above included such issues as mass storage devices, graphics hardware and accelerators, network adapters, multimedia I/O devices, and compression/decompression extensions (see figure 1.3).

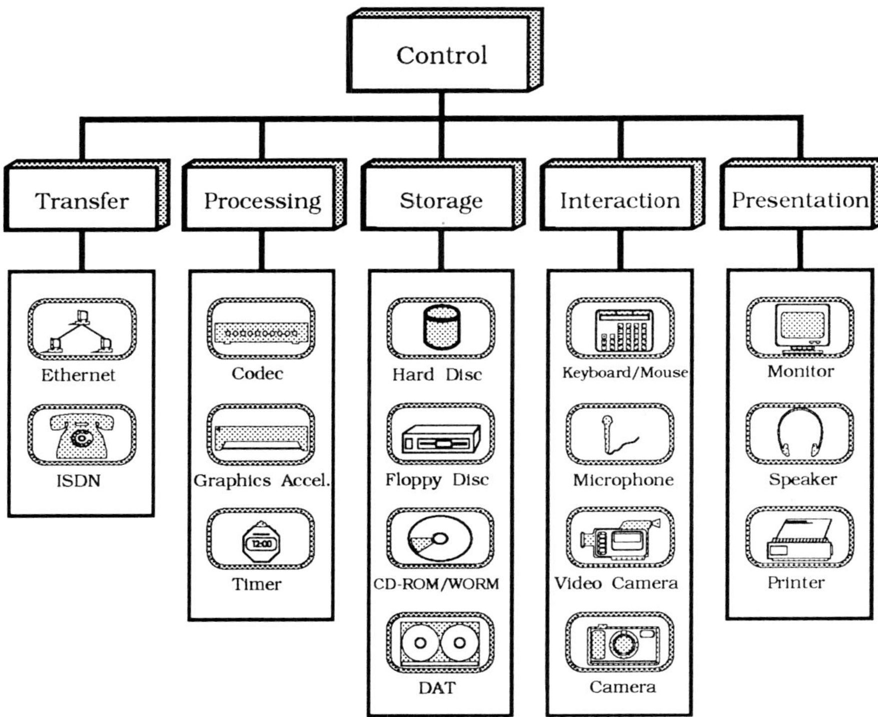

Fig 1.3. Extended hardware requirements of a CHM Workstation

Our main goal was to develop a multi-platform and multimedia communication framework for networked multimedia workstations and applications within a reasonable cost-to-quality range. Consequently, we decided to use the TCP/IP network protocol for all our implementations. Originally, TCP/IP was not designed to provide real-time communication capabilities but is a widely accepted standard. In contrast to our approach of using well established network standards, other working groups, like the Tenet Group [5, 6] or the IBM HeiTS project group [7], are currently working on new network and transport layer protocols for real-time multimedia communication.

For the operating system and the graphical user interface the choice was again heterogeneous:

- UNIX/X11/Motif on Sun Sparc and SGI Indigo
- DOS/Windows 3.1 (Windows NT) including the multimedia extensions on PCs

The support of such heterogeneous hardware and software platforms resulted in different problems concerning local process communication on each computer platform, and global process communication over the network.

These problems were solved by either using common standards and protocols (such as TCP/IP, Berkeley Sockets, graphics exchange formats, text formats) or by adapting individual mechanisms to a higher level protocol (for example local process communication was implemented using Shared Memory on the Sparc and Indigo, Dynamic Data Exchange on the PC).

Two standard network technologies are used. Ethernet as our Local Area Network and Basic Rate ISDN as our Wide Area Network. Ethernet-to-ISDN bridges are incorporated to permit such connectivity.

2 Projects and Test Platforms

Models such as the CHM model and concepts such as Tele-Media cannot be developed and evaluated without a real test application and a sufficiently sizeable environment on which to exercise them. Projects including distributed computing and multimedia communication on LANs and WANs are best tested on an international scale. This helps to achieve results that can subsequently be incorporated into commercial products.

2.1 The DEDICATED Project

DEDICATED (*De*velopment of a new *Di*mension in *C*omputer *A*ssisted *T*eaching and *Ed*ucation) is a project within the European DELTA program. The project partners come from four European countries: Germany, France, Greece and Portugal.

DEDICATED's overall goal is to develop, establish and evaluate *Local Training Centres (LTCs)* as centres of local teaching expertise, and connect these centres to form a European-wide network of *Computer Based Training* (CBT) sites (see figure 2.1) [8].

An LTC will give support to three different user groups: firstly, the courseware designers and developers who produce the learning material; secondly, the teachers and learners who deliver the courses and use the material; and thirdly, the administrators and managers who run and control the LTCs. To support these different and heterogeneous user groups, a carefully designed architecture with well defined interfaces is necessary. In DEDICATED, a hierarchical structure is proposed consisting of a generic learning server, dedicated learning tools and modular course elements.

DEDICATED's courses are based on multimedia contents and allow co-operative work and remote access. The interoperability between heterogeneous LTC platforms, and the portability of tools, course elements and whole courses are therefore substantial goals.

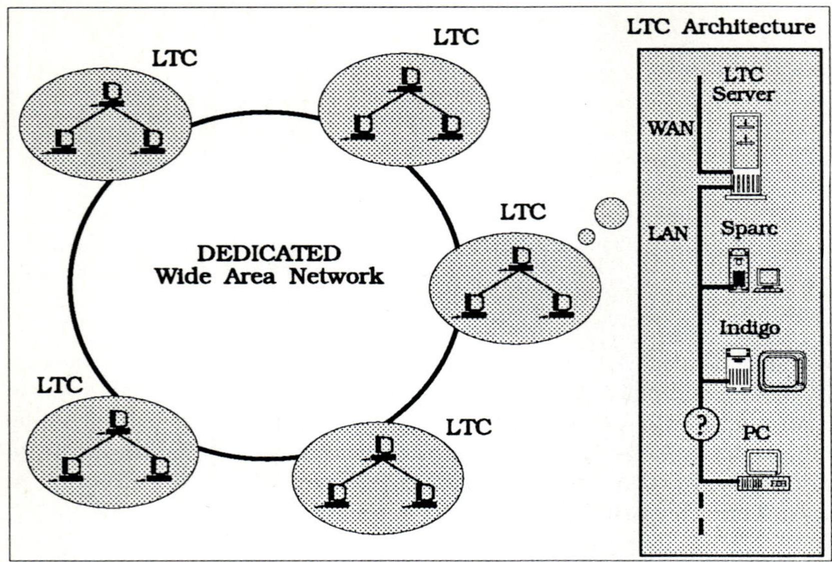

Fig. 2.1. DEDICATED's LTC architecture

As part of the R&D phase of DEDICATED, the user's needs will be constantly tracked and reports given to the R&D groups. This will help identify and correct shortcomings within DEDICATED, and hence influence the development of a long-term strategy for European-wide CBT.

The DEDICATED environment supports four learning scenarios:

1. stand alone learning
2. interactive teaching
3. lecturing
4. group learning

For each of these scenarios, Tele-Media need to be applied in order to provide multimedia learning support [9].

2.2 CHM platform CoMEdiA

CoMEdiA (*Co*-operative hyper*M*edia *Edi*ting *A*rchitecture) enables a group of 1 to 6 co-authors to co-operatively produce CHM documents. It allows co-authors to communicate their ideas and exchange information (remotely or face-to-face) until a final CHM document is achieved [10, 11].

CoMEdiA is Motif-based (see figure 2.2) and exploits a distributed client-server mechanism. Many of the CoMEdiA features can be applied to the

DEDICATED learning environment, especially those concerning co-operation and communication needs which can be extended to allow teachers and students to exchange information over long distances. CoMEdiA provides both content-based media (text, pixel-images and 2D-graphics), and communication based Tele-Media (text, audio and video). Moreover, both personal and shared text, video and voice annotations are supported.

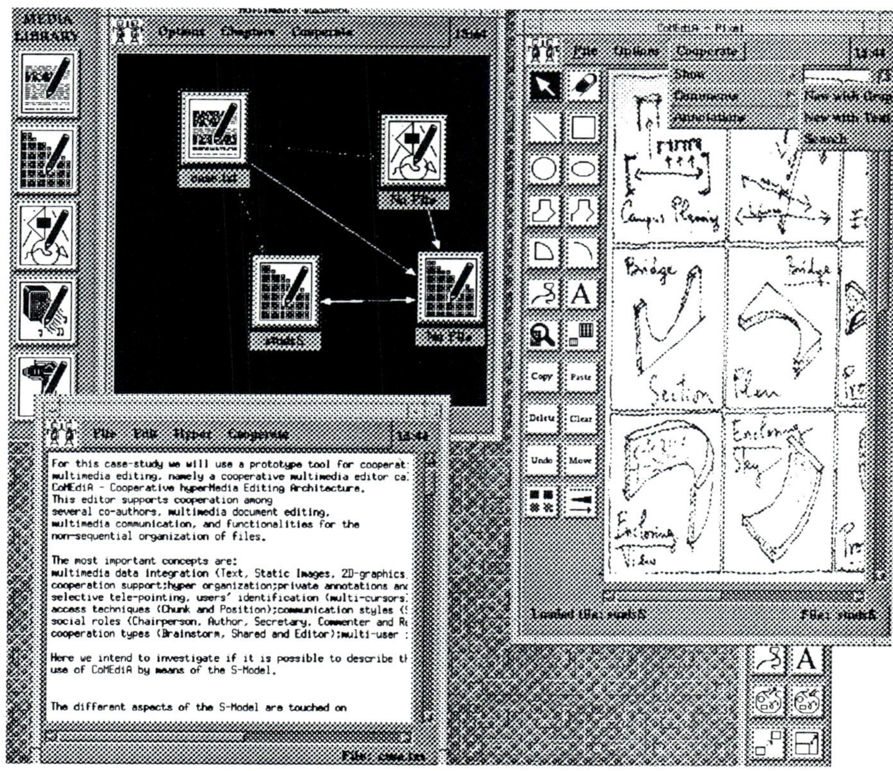

Fig. 2.2. A part of the CoMEdiA desktop (Source: A. Santos, A. Marcos)

3 Generic Tools for Real-Time Communication

Today, the concept of people at distant locations communicating with each other both visually and verbally over a telephone line (otherwise known as video conferencing) has become a reality in meeting rooms and on desktops. Video conferencing has been technically possible for years [12], but at such great cost that it was a practical alternative for only large organisations with specially designed facilities (Bellcore, NTT, Xerox). Nowadays, The use of universal multimedia standards and improvements in Workstation technology have led to much smaller systems with lower costs. These developments have made desktop multimedia affordable.

3.1 Video

Although the technology for videoconferencing has become cheaper and more powerful, the same cannot be said for communication devices. The very fast FDDI network technology can be used but is very expensive so it is necessary to use compression if we wish to manage real-time video and audio data (see figure 3.1).

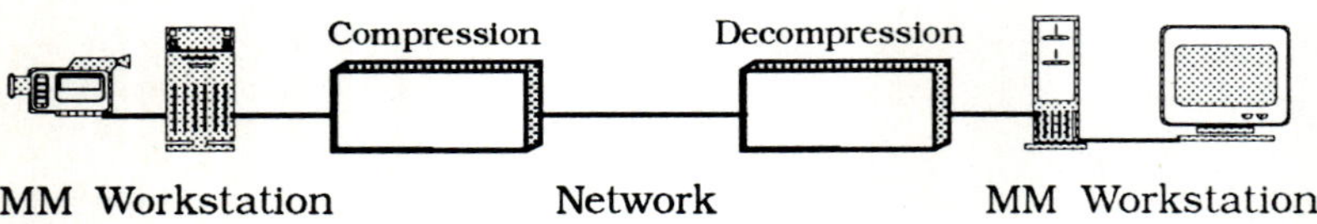

Fig. 3.1. Real-time video connection between workstations

Video compression and decompression (codec) is one area of technology currently receiving a great amount of attention. The *MPEG* (Moving Pictures Expert Group) [13] or *H.261* [14, 15] standards for video compression could have been used within this project. These codec algorithms do inter frame compression where an image in a video sequence is handled with regard to previous and succeeding images. For a given compression ratio these techniques provide a very high quality sequence of images, but are much more costly to encode and do not provide easy access to single images of the sequence.

For our system we needed a faster codec algorithm that could be performed in real-time on low-end hardware or in software, and which provided easy access to single images. The real-time issues for video as a communication channel were more important than high quality pixel and colour resolution. So we decided to use the *JPEG* (Joint Photographic Expert Group) codec [16] standard for our video frames, calling it *M-JPEG* (Motion-JPEG). This codec algorithm does a pure intra frame compression which means that it compresses a single image at a time, without regard to the previous or succeeding image.

Our prototype uses VideoPix hardware on Sun workstations, IndigoVideo on SGI workstations, and miroMovie and MISTER COOL capture hardware on PCs. VideoPix, IndigoVideo and miroMovie are commercial frame grabbers. *MISTER COOL* (*M*ultimedia *IS*DN *Ter*minal for *Co*-operation over *L*ong distances) is a PC-based low-cost hardware system that comprises a frame grabber and codec unit for transmitting video images over low-bandwidth networks [17].

The original resolution of our individual digital video image is given by the PAL video standard. These images are then reduced to 176x144 pixels with 16 grey scales, following the H.261 (Px64) specification for the image size [12, 13]. Other operation modes supported by our prototype use 352x288 pixels (resolution of the Common Intermediate Format - CIF) or 176x144 pixels (resolution of the Quarter Common Intermediate Format - QCIF) with 128 grey scales or 160 colours [16].

On a PC equipped with a MISTER COOL extension the M-JPEG codec algorithm is implemented in hardware. The resolution of the transmitted video is 176x144 pixels with 16 grey scales per pixel and a frame rate of 8.33 per second. The codec algorithm is optimised to achieve precisely the same data rate as one ISDN channel, 64 kilobits per second [17]. An extended M-JPEG video communication was implemented on UNIX workstations. The codec algorithm is realised as a software solution for Sun Sparc 2/10 and Silicon Graphics Indigo workstations. The frame grabber hardware is machine-dependent (VideoPix, IndigoVideo).

One of the main features of our prototype is the manipulation of a set of codec parameters [18]. The goal was to enable the application (or the user) to work in a flexible space, selecting parameters for image quality, frame rate, compression and decompression speed, colour mode, image size and so on. All this scalability is implemented and it has been possible to observe interesting results and new ideas for future developments.

With the Motif-based software-only solution, the frame rate is approximately 4 to 5 frames per second on a Sun Sparc 2. Therefore, the MISTER COOL PC theoretically can provide data at a faster rate than the Workstation can handle. Consequently, the Workstation does not necessarily decompress all of the incoming video frames or the PC does only send a fraction of the possible frame number.

The number of decompressed frames per second on the receiving Workstation is dependent of its CPU load. Interpolating additional frames from existing, decompressed ones and inserting them between the original frames is less CPU power consuming than decompressing frames. Therefore interpolation increases the frame rate on the Workstation and allows cross-platform adaptation (see 1.2 - Tele-Media). This mechanism is called *I*ntermediate *I*mage *I*nterpolation (I^3) and is represented in figure 3.2. As a result of the implemented I^3 mechanism, the frame rate is doubled at very reasonable computing costs without additional network usage [3, 18].

On the receiving machine, one frame is displayed on the screen and the next (decompressed) frame taken from the network and stored in a Network Frame Buffer. An interpolated version of these two original frames is calculated and saved in the Intermediate Frame Buffer. The interpolated frame is then copied to the display buffer and displayed on the monitor. When the next frame from the network has been decompressed, the preceding frame is copied from the Network Frame Buffer to the display and the new frame is stored in its place. Then the cycle starts again, interpolating between the two stored frames.

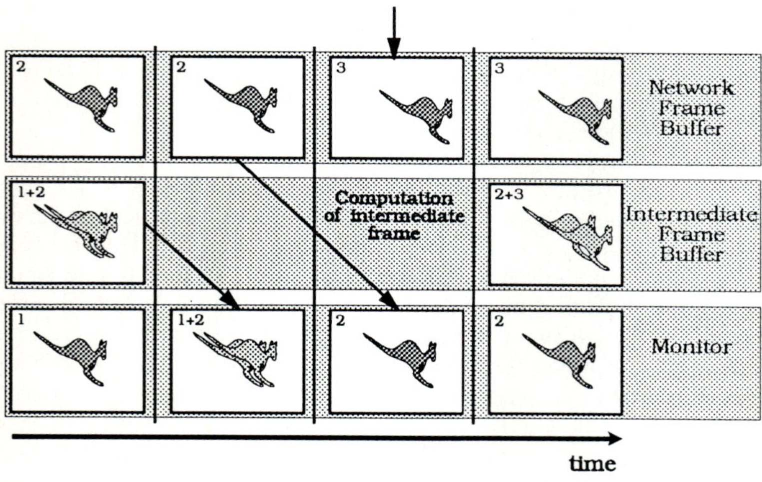

Fig. 3.2 The Intermediate Image Interpolation scheme

In our prototype tested on a Sun Sparc 2, the currently most significant limiting factor is the access time to the frame grabber hardware. With the VideoPix hardware, it takes about three times longer to grab the video data than to compress them. Therefore, within the current prototype, the video performance is not higher than 4 to 5 images/sec. Here the network is not the limiting factor because the amount of transmitted data is within the 64 Kbits/sec range.

As a conclusion we can state that, by using faster frame grabber hardware and new-generation workstations, reasonable video frame rates could be reached in practice. This is true for both the sending and receiving of video images simultaneously because the M-JPEG codec algorithms are symmetric.

3.2 Audio

Perhaps the most important -- and often overlooked -- component of video conferencing is that of audio, which can easily be lost in the coding/decoding shuffle. Surprisingly, most complaints about video conferencing are related to audio quality [3], perhaps because 60% of the information transmitted during a video conference is verbal and therefore people notice when such an important information source is degraded.

Different multimedia platforms provide different types of audio devices and services. Nevertheless, all of them offer a common set of functionalities, like record, store and playback. We realised on-line Tele-Media speech communication, using these basic functionalities. In order to provide cross-platform usability, we defined a common, *intermediate exchange format* and realised a number of on-line bi-directional converters supporting different audio formats.

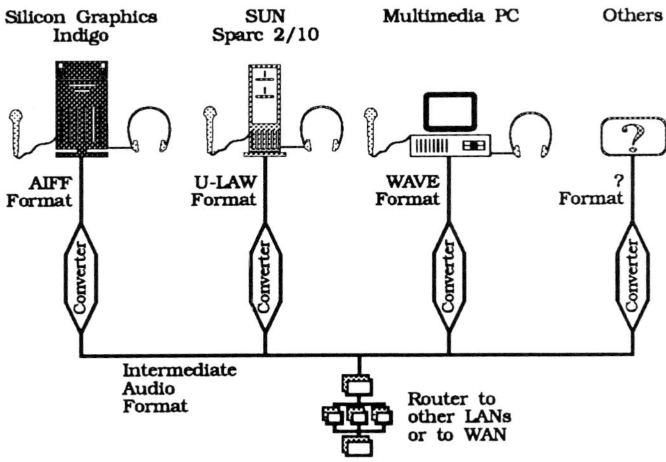

Fig. 3.3. The real-time audio connection between CHM workstations

In our system, we provide a number of on-line converters to support different audio formats:

- U-LAW for Sun workstations
- AIFF for SGI workstations
- WAVE for Multimedia PCs

Our intermediate exchange format used for all platforms is a subset of the WAVE format. The reason for the choice of the WAVE format was its simplicity and the superior processing speed of the converters on Sun and Silicon Graphic workstations in comparison to converters on the PC. On the workstations the converters only produce delays of approximately 12.5 milliseconds each. The Multimedia PC accepts the intermediate WAVE format without any conversion which results in reduced computational costs. The WAVE format as used on our prototype is based on the *Pulse Code Modulated* (PCM) data format of 8-bit mono at a sample rate of 8 kHz (voice-quality). It can reproduce a limited dynamic range of the human voice. The audio transfer rate sums up to 64 Kbits/sec, what is precisely the data rate of one ISDN channel.

On occasions it might be useful to record the exchanged audio data during a tele-conferencing session, for later playback, for archiving issues or for editing. But even voice-quality audio is data intensive; one minute of voice quality audio takes almost half a Mbyte of storage space. Therefore, on-line codec algorithms to minimise storage space and network bandwidth are needed, covering both the raw data and precise timing information such as sample rate, recording time and synchronisation markers.

We realised mechanisms called *up-sampling* and *down-sampling*. They allow very fast changes of the sample rate of the transmitted and processed audio data without modifying the used audio hardware. Down-sampling means that a part of the audio samples on the sender side are discarded before transmitting the audio stream and broadcasting the "new" sample rate. If down-sampling from 8 kHz to 4 kHz is selected every second sample is discarded. The up-sampling algorithm on the receiver side restores the audio signal either to its original sample rate or to some other selected sample rate. This is done by interpolating the missing audio samples from the existing data and is very similar to the I^3 mechanism introduced in 3.1 - Video. These mechanisms might be used both for reducing the transmitted data and for the *cross-platform adaptation* of two different audio systems. Even with a transmitted sample rate of 4 kHz the quality of sound is good enough for communication purposes.

So as not to overload the network, we introduced a *noise gate*. Just voice above a certain volume level gets transmitted, but not the background noise during the times when no one is speaking, or the microphone is switched off. As with the on-line converters, the noise gate is realised using software on the workstations. The delay during the audio data transmission produced by the noise gate is less than 7.5 milliseconds on Sun or Silicon Graphics workstations, dependent on the processing load. The on-line converters consume less than 12.5 milliseconds each. This totals a worst case delay of approximately 30 milliseconds for the entire conversion, not taking into account the delays due to the physical network. The audio data rate is always less than 64 Kbits/sec which can be easily provided by LANs or ISDN.

3.3 Synchronising Audio and Video

We implemented combined audio/video mechanisms in order to reach media synchronisation to maximise human comprehension. We have been defining an *Integrated Format for Audio and Video* (IFAV), that provides audio and video data in AV Frames (Audio/Video Frames). Each AV Frame includes one or more video frames (compressed or uncompressed), the audio data belonging to the video frames, and exact timing information in order to allow both synchronity and isochronity of the IFAV data stream.

The IFAV mechanisms developed can be used to implement cross-platform audio/video communication functionalities based on the Audio Video Interleaf (AVI), QuickTime or Minimal Video Extension to X (MVEX) standards [19, 20, 21]. The underlying Tele-Media-based mechanisms are supposed to reduce the number of transmitted or displayed video images in situations where the video bandwidth is decreased but the audio data stream or the synchronity between audio and video must be maintained. The primary goal is to realise smart audio/video communication mechanisms that are self-adaptable to changing system capabilities.

A first prototype is already in the testing phase providing experience with our synchronisation mechanisms and IFAV format. The formats for the audio and the video data streams are the same as with the individual real-time Tele-Media audio and video. We can already record and playback audio/video sequences allowing isochronity.

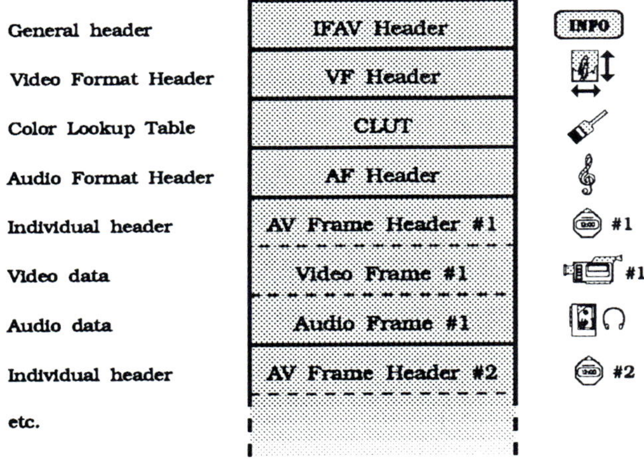

Fig. 3.4. The IFAV file format; it contains general information about file size and media formats, special video and audio information, a colour look-up table if necessary, timing information, and audio and video data.

4 Future Plans

We have already implemented a system that allows multimedia communication on heterogeneous and distributed platform. The near future will bring the integration of new features.

- The network communication between workstations and PCs will be extended.
- Windows NT will be supported.
- In order to support more advanced audio codec mechanism we are planning to implement the ADPCM (Adaptive Differential Pulse Code Modulation) algorithm for our intermediate exchange format. This will allow a codec rate of 2 to 3 with much better audio quality. Moreover, we want to include a low-pass filter in order to reduce audio aliasing effects.
- We are also planning to use the Integrated Format for Audio and Video (IFAV) for communication purposes when strict synchronity (lip synchronisation) is needed. Therefore we will develop more sophisticated cross-platform timer mechanisms.
- We want to merge the IFAV and the Video for Windows (AVI) mechanisms.
- Multicast/multipoint communication mechanisms allowing more than two user to communicate simultaneously are currently in a test phase and will be extended in the future.

All these new features will be tested and evaluated within the DEDICATED and CoMEdiA projects. This will give the necessary feedback and expertise to develop elaborate co-operative multimedia applications with extended real-time communication features and will also influence standardisation work.

5 Conclusion

The CHM model of co-operative access, hypermedia organisation and multimedia content is future-oriented, but many facets of it are already being realised.

The multimedia desktop Workstation is the *communication centre* of the future. Towards the end of this century, information must be accessible in many forms. Personal and co-operative multimedia on heterogeneous, networked workstations provides interactive co-operation among distributed users who are sharing their knowledge and expertise over long distances. Right now, we are at the beginning of a new era of information management and distribution which could well change our society as dramatically as telephone technology only a few decades ago; the centre of a new technology is not the *man-machine interface*, but the *human-to-human interface*.

The concept of Tele-Media presented here and its first implementation in a heterogeneous, distributed and co-operative learning environment marks a step towards future more human-oriented computer and network systems.

Acknowledgement

We thank Prof. J. Encarnação for the opportunities and suggestions given; A. Santos, A. Marcos and M. Jäger for the support given and the fruitful discussions; O. Eichhorn, A. S. Vieira and R. Worsch for their help in the implementation; and Dr. V. Burrill for proof-reading this paper.

References

1. Ch. Hornung, M. Jaeger, A. Santos, B. Tritsch, "Cooperative HyperMedia - An Enabling Paradigm for Cooperative Work", *The Visual Computing Special Issue on "Techniques and Applications of Computer Graphics in the Context of Telecommunications"*, 1993 (in press)
2. E. Fox, "Multimedia: Application and Practice", *Tutorial Notes: Eurographics 92*, Cambridge, September 1992
3. A. Santos, B. Tritsch, "Using Multimedia to Support Cooperative Editing", as accepted at the *Eurographics '93*, Barcelona, September 1993
4. R. Steinmetz, "Synchronization Properties in Multimedia Systems", *IEEE Journal on Selected Areas in Communications, Vol. 8, No. 3, pp. 401-412*, April 1990
5. A. Banerjea, B. A. Mah, "The Real-Time Channel Administration Protocol", The Tenet Group, *Proc. 2nd Intl. Workshop on Network and Operating System Support for Digital Audio and Video, Lecture Notes in Computer Science, No. 614, pp. 160-170*, Heidelberg, Nov. 1991
6. D. Ferrari, "Design and Applications of a Delay Jitter Control Scheme for Packet-Switching Internetworks", The Tenet Group, *Proc. 2nd Intl. Workshop on Network and Operating System Support for Digital Audio and Video, Lecture Notes in Computer Science, No. 614, pp. 72-83*, Heidelberg, Nov. 1991
7. R. Steinmetz, Th. Meyer, "Modelling Distributed Multimedia Applications", IBM European Networking Center, Heidelberg
8. Brisson-Lopes, Gomes, Graf, Knierriem, Lindner, Tritsch, Velez, Zysk, "Functional Specification of the Modular Training System", *DELTA Deliverable 3, Project D2014 DEDICATED*, DELTA Commission of the European Community, August 1992
9. B. Tritsch, Ch. Hornung, "DEDICATED - Learning on Networked Multimedia Platforms", as accepted at the *IFIP Working Conference on Visualization in Scientific Computing: Uses in University Education*, Irvine, California, July 1993
10. A. Santos, "CoMEdiA: Conceptualization and Realization of a Cooperative HyperMedia Editing Architecture", *Second Eurographics Workshop on Multimedia*, Darmstadt, May 1992
11. A. Santos, A. Marcos, "An Algorithm and Architecture to Support Cooperative Multimedia Editing", as accepted at the *4th Workshop on Future Trends in Distributed Computing Systems*, Lisbon, September 1993
12. S. Gale, "Desktop Video Conferencing: Technical Advances and Evaluation Issues", *Computer Communications, Vol. 15, No. 8, pp. 512-526*, 1992
13. D. LeGall, "MPEG: A Video Compression Standard for Multimedia Applications", *Communications of the ACM, Vol. 34, No. 4, pp 46-58*, 1991
14. "Video Codec for Audiovisual Services at Px64 kBits/s", *CCITT Rec. H.261, CDM XV-R 37E*, CCITT, August 1990
15. M. Liou, "Overview of the Px64 Kbit/s Video Coding Standard"; *Communications of the ACM 34, 4 (1991), pp. 59-63*, 1991
16. "JPEG Technical Specification", *Joined Photographic Expert Group ISO/IEC, JTC1/SC2/WG8*, CCITT SGVIII, August 1989

17. M. Jaeger, B. Tritsch, "Multimedia in a Tele-Cooperative Environment - Performing Video on an ISDN-PC", *Proc. of the 2nd Eurographics Workshop on Multimedia, pp. 127-138*, May 1992

18. B. Tritsch, A. S. Vieira, Ch. Hornung, " Video and Audio Communication over LAN", as accepted at the *IFIP Working Conference on The Open System Future: Leveraging the LAN*, Perth, August 1993

19. CCETT, "Multimedia Synchronization", *CCETT Int. note: AFNOR adhoc group on AVI standardization*, July 1988

20. D. Littman, T. Moran, "QuickTime: It's about time", *Mac World, pp 80-81*, August 1991

21. T. Brunhoff, "MVEX Slides", *X Conference '92*, 1992

Distributed Multimedia Solutions from the HeiProjects

Ralf Guido Herrtwich

IBM European Networking Center
Vangerowstraße 18 • 69115 Heidelberg • Germany

rgh @ dhdibmip.bitnet

Abstract: The HeiProjects are aimed at providing a universal multimedia platform for networked workstations. This platform shall be used to support distributed multimedia applications, e.g., for collaboration support or multimedia kiosks. Its core component is a multimedia transport system spanning several underlying communication networks with different degrees of multimedia support. This paper provides a survey of the system together with proposed solutions for individual components as they appear from today's perspective.

1 Introduction

Most existing multimedia products today are constrained to local, stand-alone computers. Many of them are only able to handle a single stream of multimedia data at a time. They are unsuitable for the more complex distributed environment that is common in businesses today.

The IBM European Networking Center (ENC) works on making distributed multimedia computing a reality. Named after the ENC location in Heidelberg, the so-called "HeiProjects" provide distributed multimedia solutions for networked kiosk installations, collaboration support, or multimedia data retrieval. These applications are built on top of a multimedia transport system spanning several underlying communication networks with different degrees of multimedia support.

This paper provides a survey of the system to be developed together with a survey of proposed solutions for individual components as they appear from today's perspective. The intention of this paper is to give the reader a first idea of our scope of work, we will not explain details. In this introduction we describe the overall structure of the system we develop as well as the fundamental beliefs and constraints underlying our work.

1.1 Distributed Multimedia – The Big Picture

Multimedia is at the focal point of information and communication technology [Fox 1991a, 1991b; Davies, Nicol 1991; Herrtwich, Steinmetz 1991]. It combines the audiovisual power of television, the publishing power of the printing press, and the interactive power of the computer. Apart from applications in education and merchandising, multimedia technology will be pervasive to the business desktop in future offices. Here, the communication functions to exchange multimedia documents and to engage in audiovisual communication are most urgently needed. The prototype development of distributed multimedia applications today offers a market advantage for the future [IBM 1991].

How could such a future look like? We envision multimedia to support scenarios such as the following:

> A chemical corporation with headquarters in Cologne has recently acquired a plant for fertilizers in Leipzig. In Cologne, one of the company's environmental officers sits at her multimedia workstation and browses through a proposal for the plant restructuring which was submitted to her by the leader of the plant reorganization task force from Leipzig.
>
> From her workstation, she first calls her secretary to provide her with the latest set of legal emission levels for Saxony. Using a graphical environment simulation tool, she checks which effect the proposed plant extension has on the emission of toxic fumes. By the time the simulation is done, her secretary has mailed the chart she requested. She finds out that the proposed plan violates the environment protection laws of Saxony. She copies the results of her simulation, adds some spoken comments to it, and sends it all back to Leipzig through multimedia mail.
>
> In Leipzig, the task force leader sees that he has to take immediate action to modify his plans. From his workstation, he calls a video conference with all other task force members. He informs the others about the legal restrictions by showing them the simulation results he got from Cologne together with the voice annotations. One task force member proposes to get in touch with one of the company's chief engineers to discuss whether they can add filters to some of the plant's reactors.
>
> The engineer is not in his office in Cologne, but can be contacted in Hamburg where another plant is under construction. He says that he cannot immediately work on the problem, but that he will get back to the task force later. He asks them to mail all their relevant documents to him. The task force leader closes the conference and sends the mail on which he has highlighted some figures to the engineer's mailbox.
>
> Later during the day, the engineer logs onto his home workstation from Hamburg and checks the material provided. He browses through catalogs of filter equipment and indeed comes to a new solution. He forwards the proposal to the financial analyst assigned to the project with the request to forward it to the task force if it is economically feasible.

This example illustrates that multimedia networking is an essential step for making multimedia technology attractive to a larger community of users. The integrated provision of audio and video to support common office procedures provides an added value to the user which justifies the expenses for new multimedia workstation equipment.

To record and playback multimedia data across geographical distances enables new services such as to arrange a private newscast from the news clips on a remote server, to set up a video conference among colleagues in different continents, or to simply call home from work using the computer. While distributed multimedia systems, on one hand, limit the need for travel through collaboration tools, on the other hand, they can make it easier for users abroad to touch base with their home office.

While communication services are essential for the introduction of multimedia in a computing environment, future multimedia applications will require advances in other areas of technology, too.

- The first generation of multimedia systems will enable media recording, exchange, and playback. This is the generation of multimedia systems our current projects are aimed at.
- The second generation will add media production. Research on virtual reality to provide realistic computer animation and sound is already underway [Krueger 1991; Rheingold 1991].
- The third generation of multimedia systems will finally provide media understanding through image and sound recognition. It would be able to accomplish tasks such as to find all sequences in Casablanca where Humphrey Bogart wears a trench-coat and talks to Ingrid Bergman, or to substitute Anne-Sophie Mutter's by Nigel Kennedy's interpretation of Vivaldi's Four Seasons in a Berlin Philharmonics' recording.

Only at this point – not within the next decade – the goal of complete media integration is achieved.

1.2 Fundamental Beliefs

Underlying the multimedia work in the HeiProjects are a set of fundamental beliefs to guide the multimedia research activities. These guidelines determine the purpose of multimedia as follows:

- First and foremost, multimedia is a set of technologies to broaden the bandwidth of perception and presentation at the man-machine interface of any kind of computer system – to make such a system more appealing and useful for humans.
- Second, multimedia enables new applications where the generality of the computer is applied to audio and motion video. It makes these media available for interactive use and free manipulation from the desktop.

While others see multimedia as an add-on technology to open up new application domains for the computer industry, we trust that multimedia will affect all areas of computing. Support for multimedia should, therefore, be inherent to all future computer systems. Multimedia system design should take into account the following principles:

- A multimedia system should be limited by performance constraints only, not by logical design. In principle, all appropriate functions applicable to traditional media should also be applicable to audio and video. In particular, this calls for the use of digital encoding of multimedia data (see also [Anderson et al. 1991]).
- Today's computing environments are distributed. Multimedia technology needs to be used in this network environment to facilitate interpersonal communication and collaborative computing.

In particular this last point leads us to pursue multimedia technology from the ENC's background in networking.

1.3 Platforms

There are two major system platforms for the HeiProjects: IBM's RS/6000 workstations and PS/2 personal computers. Additional work is done for PCs and Apple Macintoshes. This means that heterogeneity is built into any project deliverable from the ground up.

The audiovisual attachments available for these system lines during the project span will be used to connect cameras, microphones, and speakers to each station. It is not intended to develop new audio or video I/O hardware as part of our effort. This means that off-the-shelf equipment (existing monitors, existing cameras, etc.) will be used.

To introduce multimedia in an particular environment, it is essential to provide audio and video facilities as evolutionary extensions of the existing system platforms. It is an obvious goal to try to change existing systems as little as possible to include multimedia. However, the different characteristics of audio and video (in particular their real-time requirements) make some changes inevitable. To achieve openness in these changes, the HeiProjects work will take into account not only existing, but also evolving industrial and international standards.

1.4 The HeiProjects

The HeiProjects are designed as a project framework to develop distributed multimedia system components. Currently, the following projects constitute the major share of the HeiProjects activities:

- The core of the HeiProjects currently is the realization of a transport system that permits the exchange of multimedia data with end-to-end performance guarantees over several networks.
- As part of the transport system development, several support functions have been identified that need to be part of any local multimedia platform.
- A toolkit shall be designed which encompasses a set of basic multimedia services for constructing distributed multimedia applications. Whereas the transport system is responsible for real-time data transfer, the toolkit provides service elements to organize and control communication.
- In the fourth category, all multimedia applications are collected. Of course, the number of possible applications is unbounded. Some applications will be realized in the HeiProjects for demonstration purposes. We also participate in the design of multimedia teleservices. In our terminology, these services are distributed multimedia applications provided in a unified form on a variety of system platforms to a large user community – akin to traditional telephone or telex services. Examples of such services are audiovisual conferencing or video-on-demand services.

A simple example can be used to illustrate the relationship between these system components. Figure 1 illustrates the retrieval of a remote video clip. This distributed application involves two application-level modules, a video client and a video server, built on top of the toolkit services. The client communicates with the server to select and to start a video. It can use traditional communication protocols for this purpose because such control operations are not time-critical.

The start request causes the server to get in touch with its local multimedia environment to start the flow of the video stream. The environment manages multimedia I/O modules termed stream handlers. One such stream handler would retrieve the data from a file, another would send it out on the network. This network stream handler for multimedia is the multimedia transport system. It uses a real-time communication protocol to transfer audio and video data.

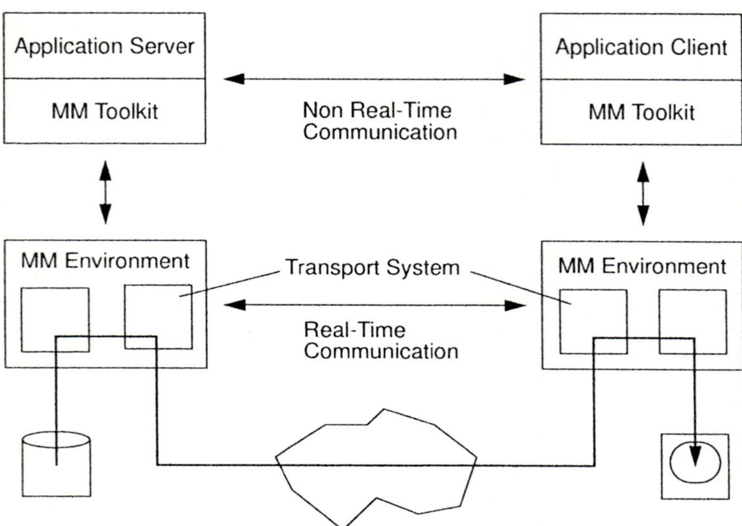

Figure 1: Sample system structure

1.5 Outline of This Document

The different multimedia system components and their constituents are described in the remainder of the document. Section 2 describes the main components of a local multimedia environment. Section 3 describes the multimedia transport system. Section 4 gives an outlook on the basic toolkit service elements to construct distributed multimedia applications. Section 5 discusses elementary multimedia applications and Section 6 introduces some multimedia teleservices.

2 Local Multimedia Environments

To design a local multimedia system is a prerequisite for achieving distributed multimedia services. In contrast to multimedia protocols and application program interfaces, different vendors providing open distributed multimedia services do not necessarily have to agree on a single local system architecture. Yet, it is likely that a local multimedia architecture will influence the design of the distributed system. An example are resource reservation techniques: To achieve real-time behavior, distributed resources in the network should be reserved in just the same fashion as local resources (e.g., using the same parameter set to define service quality).

The HeiProjects are not mainly concerned with designing and implementing local multimedia services, but rather use existing work in this area and extend it if needed. Among the most prominent multimedia environments available today is IBM's Multimedia Presentation Manager/2 [IBM 1992]. MMPM/2 operates on top of multimedia device adapters such as CD-ROM drives, audio I/O cards, and video compression/decompression boards. It also provides means to program software functions to be included as filters for multimedia data.

A main function of multimedia environments such as MMPM/2 is to provide a real-time environment (RTE) to handle digital audio and video. Within this RTE, the temporal dependencies that are characteristic for presenting multimedia data to a human user are obeyed. The RTE schedules the processing of multimedia data according to the data's inherent urgency. On a multimedia computer system, the RTE coexists with a non-real-time environment (NRTE) which deals with all data that has no timing parameters associated with it. Most of today's computer systems contain an NRTE only, others provide an RTE only (e.g., in process automation). The challenge lies in the combination of both environments.

Multimedia I/O devices in general are accessed from both environments: Data such as a video frame is passed to them from the RTE, whereas control operations such as a camera zoom come from the NRTE. From an application viewpoint, the RTE is completely shielded by the NRTE: For real-time data, the application only performs control functions (it only "sets the proper switches") and is not involved in the actual data transfer. It may, however, influence the way data is handled, e.g., by inserting a filter function in the processing queue.

The main purpose of any multimedia environment is to manage the flow of multimedia data. This portion is usually termed the Stream Management Subsystem (SMS). To obey the real-time requirements of multimedia data, a Resource Management Subsystem (RMS) avoids resource overload and takes care of appropriate resource scheduling. To optimize the flow of data through the system for performance, a Buffer Management Subsystem (BMS) is used. These subsystems are described in more detail in the following sections.

2.1 Stream Management Subsystem (SMS)

Any entity handling multimedia data in the RTE is called a stream handler [Herrtwich 1992]. Typical stream handlers are filter and mixing functions, but also multimedia communication subsystems (or parts of them). Stream handlers also encapsulate multimedia I/O devices. Each stream handler has endpoints for input and/or output through which data units flow. The stream handler consumes data units from one or more input endpoints, it generates data units through one or more output endpoints.

The SMS enables applications to access stream handlers by instantiating them. Each stream handler is created for exclusive use by one application. The quality of service (QOS) a stream handler provides is determined by the RMS upon creation (see next section).

In a typical system, multimedia data flows repeatedly from output to input endpoints. The purpose of the SMS is to connect endpoints to an acyclic, unidirectional stream handler graph as shown in Figure 2. The resulting stream handler conduits[1] are either static or dynamic. Static conduits are predefined and cannot be modified by applications. Statically connected stream handlers appear to the application as one single stream handler. In the transport system one can, e.g., statically connect network and transport layer software although each software module may constitute a stream handler in its own right. Dynamic conduits are created by the application through corresponding *connect* and *disconnect* functions. For example, the connection of a transport system stream handler to a display stream handler is dynamic.

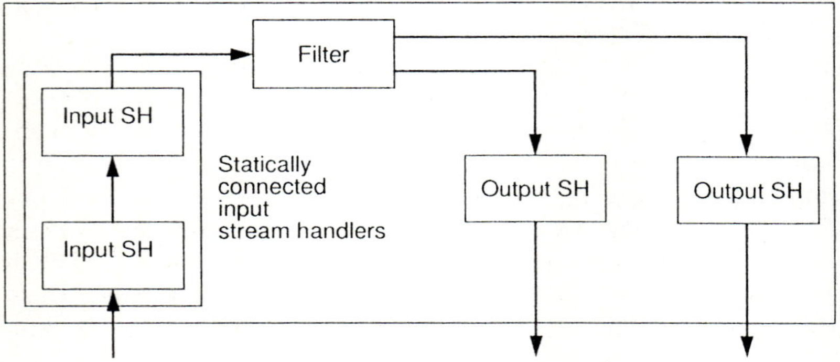

Figure 2: A stream handler graph.

Once a connection is established, multimedia data flows directly from one stream handler into another within the RTE. The data is usually not passed to the application; should the application require copies of the data it may obtain them on request. As entering the application involves leaving the RTE, the multimedia data looses its temporal properties in this case.

Within the RTE, the SMS provides the function of stream synchronization. Synchronization is specified on a conduit basis. Any conduit may be synchronized to avoid jitter, but usually synchronization will be used only for conduits to sinks; only here the synchronization is apparent to the human user [Ferrari 1991]. Synchronization can be expressed using the notions of "clocks" or "logical time systems" [Anderson, Homsy 1991; Herrtwich 1991b]. These abstractions serve as a reference system to determine time points at which the processing of data units shall commence.

1. The term "conduit" is used to distinguish connections between stream handlers from network connections.

2.2 Resource Management Subsystem (RMS)

Whenever a stream handler is created, a certain quality of service (QOS) is associated with it. To negotiate this QOS between the system and the application is the purpose of the RMS. The RMS relies on appropriate resource scheduling techniques to maintain an agreed-on QOS [Herrtwich 1991a]. Within the HeiProjects, a special resource management method called HeiRAT, the Heidelberg Resource Administration Technique, has been developed [Vogt, Herrtwich, Nagarajan 1992].

Providing a certain QOS involves reserving some fraction of an underlying (hardware) resource to guarantee the availability of the necessary bandwidth to accomplish this service. Two basic QOS classes can be distinguished:

- Guaranteed (or pessimistic) QOS is based on the assumption that a drop of service quality has to be avoided. Therefore, a resource reservation for the worst case is made.
- Best-effort (or optimistic) QOS assumes that a few QOS conflicts may occur and can be handled by the application. In this case, reservations are only made for the average or minimum workload.

Best-effort QOS achieves a better utilization of the underlying resource at the expense of service quality. It should be chosen if resource capacity is scarce and maximum and average workload differ significantly.

The QOS parameters used in HeiRAT include throughput and delay. Throughput is specified in terms of the maximum, average, or minimum size of logical data units (e.g., audio access units or video frames) and the rate of these logical data units. Delay is defined by minimum and maximum transit time of logical data units (also defining jitter bounds for delivering a data unit).

QOS parameters are always negotiated between the system and the application. An application may either provide values for all QOS parameters as input for this negotiation, or it may leave one parameter open for optimization by the RMS (e.g., for a certain throughput, the shortest delay shall be determined).

Simple QOS negotiation procedures determine a QOS when a stream handler is created and maintain it throughout the stream handler's existence. Adaptive QOS negotiation schemes try to balance the QOS provided and the number of applications satisfied [Hanko et al. 1991]. The more stream handlers are created, the lower the QOS for each of them will be. To the application, adaptive QOS negotiation leads to a gracefully degrading service; it may require the application to use smaller audio sampling rates or worse image resolution. Best-effort stream handlers provide the starting point for implementing adaptive procedures. They are also useful to support multi-party applications where individual parties can tolerate different service qualities.

2.3 Buffer Management Subsystem (BMS)

Handling digital multimedia data with good image and sound quality pushes the abilities of today's workstations to the limit. The single most important performance factor in piping multimedia data through the workstation is the amount of physical data movement that has to take place – both in regard to the amount of interrupts initiating a copy operation and the volume of data to be copied. The BMS has the task to minimize such movements. It inserts only those move or copy operations that are physically required by the machine architecture.

The HeiProjects have designed their own Heidelberg Buffer Management System, HeiBMS [McKellar 1993]. It provides a flat memory space for non-uniform semiconductor storage. It can access data both in main memory and on an adapter. In the ideal case, data is moved from the memory of a multimedia input device adapter straight across the bus to the output adapter. If such a transfer is not possible (either because an adapter is not capable of gaining bus control or because the data formats of input and output are not compatible and require adjustment) intermediate storage in the workstation's main memory is required. This is also needed if the workstation actually has to process the multimedia data.

HeiBMS constructs buffers from buffer fragments. Fragments of a buffer may be located at arbitrary places in the flat memory space HeiBMS controls. They are not physically aligned until data is passed to an output device. This is convenient for stream handlers which add or remove certain portions of a data unit, e.g., the time stamp of a video frame. In a layered architecture such as that of a multimedia communication system where each communication layer adds or removes headers or trailers to data units, fragment support is crucial to the system performance.

Usually, a buffer or buffer fragment is allocated somewhere in the system and then forwarded from entity to entity until it is finally removed. In some cases buffers need to be kept for later. Retransmission in a communication system is a typical example for this. HeiBMS provides locking functions for this purpose. They go hand in hand with facilities to share buffers among entities.

2.4 Operating System Independence

Technically, any system intended to run on a variety of platforms benefits from an abstraction layer that hides the differences of the underlying software as much as possible. The HeiProjects have designed such an abstraction in HeiOSS, the Heidelberg Operating System Shield. It currently provides a common interface to the main AIX and OS/2 operating system routines such as semaphore operations or timing.

3 Multimedia Transport

All forms of using multimedia in a distributed environment involve transporting multimedia data from sources to sinks. The application context determines parameters of the transport. Two dominant factors can be identified for choosing a certain transport QOS: the kind of media to be transported (different kinds of audio and video), and whether sources or sinks are multimedia I/O devices. For example, audio has more stringent requirements on delay than video and display of stored video clips leaves more freedom of scheduling than live conferencing [Hehmann et al. 1989].

HeiTS, the Heidelberg Transport System, denotes the subproject concerned with providing the facilities to transport multimedia data with different QOS requirements across a variety of underlying networks. As usual for communication systems, HeiTS follows a layered approach: It runs both a network and transport protocol on top of the underlying networks' LLC and MAC protocols. These modules are described in more detail in the following subsections.

3.1 Network Attachments

To provide multimedia services in today's typical workstation environment requires to send audio and video data across networks which were not designed for this purpose. Problems of using existing networks such as Ethernet and Token Ring are twofold: First, the networks may not provide sufficient bandwidth to carry multimedia data. Second, the networks may not be able to guarantee a certain QOS.

Bandwidth problems can most easily be overcome using new fiber networks. Then again, compression techniques for multimedia data make multimedia transport even across narrowband networks feasible, albeit with losses in data quality. The QOS problem is more difficult to handle: It requires both reservation mechanisms and the ability to control access to the reserved bandwidth (which is non-trivial if access is distributed). Bandwidth can be a brute-force solution to the QOS problem: The less scarce resource capacity is, the more likely it is that the desired QOS is maintained.

Sessions within the communication system are tantamount to connections. To reduce session administration and QOS negotiation overhead, multiplexing of connections from one layer to another should be avoided. As both multimedia and traditional data shall be sent over the same networks, a dual queueing approach becomes important: Time-critical data units are separated from non-time-critical data so that they can be given preferred service. A priority scheme is enabled for each network, with assigning highest priority to multimedia data units. Messages can be "colored", i.e., marked with their priority, to be able to distinguish them within the network to allow bridges, switches, and routers to maintain the dual queueing without requiring connection information [Nagarajan, Vogt 1992].

The set of networks to be used for HeiTS is, in principle, not limited. One important goal is the attachment of workstations to Broadband ISDN because of its expected market share in the medium term [Bocke, Armbruster 1991]. This includes the provision of a network adapter connecting IBM workstations to Broadband ISDN with ATM technology. However, internetworking between Broadband ISDN and other networks is also important as it facilitates the participation of users in multimedia services without large investments in network infrastructure.

16 Mbit/s Token Ring is our choice for a low-end multimedia network. To also include new generation local area networks, FDDI will be supported. Additional networks which lend themselves as candidates for inclusion in HeiTS are ISDN and VBN, a switched broadband network in Germany. Ethernet will also be considered. All networks together result in an internetworking structure as depicted in Figure 3.

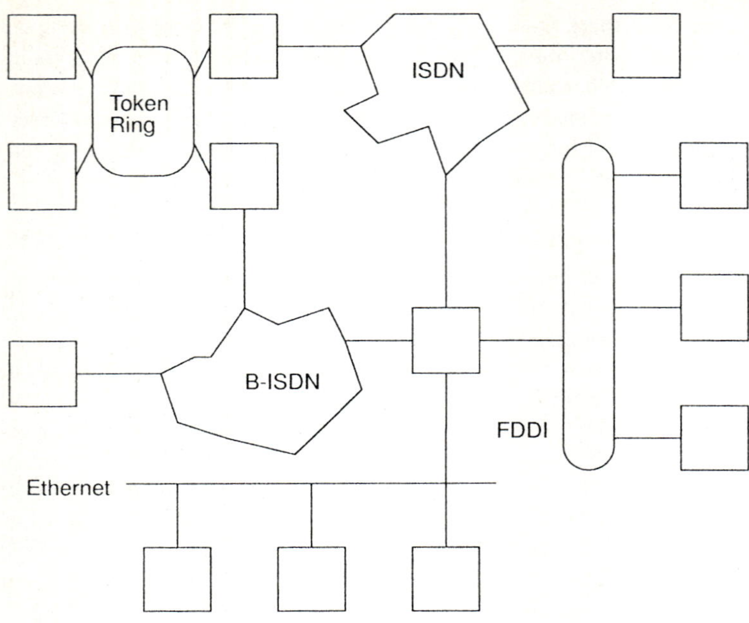

Figure 3: Internetworking with HeiTS

3.2 Data Link Layer

To make HeiTS interface with all the different networks underneath, a common data link service is implemented for all of them. HeiDL, the Heidelberg Data Link, provides the same interface for all networks. One of HeiDL's most important features is to make multicast in the underlying networks available so that it can be utilized by the protocol layers above.

HeiDL administrates multicast groups within a local network and negotiates multicast group addresses. This negotiation ensures that the multicast group address is unique so that packets are never misdelivered. HeiDL provides the facility to negotiate a Layer 2 multicast address and to map this address to a Layer 3 address. Thus, dynamic or transient multicast groups are supported. Obviously, this scheme relies on networks supporting multicast addresses. Ethernet, Token Ring, and FDDI all provide this facility.

3.3 Network Layer

The network layer is the core of HeiTS. This is where two essential multimedia communication functions are provided: multicast support as needed for audiovisual conferencing and distribution applications, and QOS negotiation for end-to-end connections.

Currently, the Internet Stream Protocol, Version II (ST-II, for short) is used to accomplish both functions [Topolcic 1990].

The elements of ST-II allow a sending origin to establish a multicast connection in the form of a routing tree to one or more receiving targets. Nodes in the tree represent ST-II agents executing the ST-II protocol, links of the tree are called hops. The origin can emit a continuous unidirectional stream of messages which are forwarded by the ST-II agents following the static routes defined by the tree. ST-II data packets are optimized for fast forwarding. This helps to keep the residence time of a packet in a particular node low and supports low-delay applications such as voice conversation.

Apart from data packets, ST-II agents exchange control packets of the ST Control Message Protocol (SCMP). SCMP serves to create, modify, and delete routing trees. As part of establishing a connection, SCMP negotiates the connection's QOS parameters. This negotiation process combines the individual QOS parameters for each resource a connection uses to an end-to-end QOS. Following the SCMP terminology, QOS parameters are collected in a flow specification of an ST-II connection.

Three kinds of entities participate in the QOS negotiation: the origin and targets as the service users, the ST-II agents, and the local HeiRAT modules as resource managers. The origin supplies an initial flow specification describing its QOS demands. This QOS request is part of a connection establishment message that is sent hop-by-hop on the paths to the targets. Each agent on such a path receiving this message calculates the QOS that the resources it controls can provide and reserves the corresponding resource capacities. These resources include capacity on the local CPU for protocol processing, local buffer space for storing messages, and bandwidth of the network.

Depending on the success of its reservations and the calculated QOS values obtained from HeiRAT (e.g., local delay), an ST-II agent updates the flow specification (e.g., keeping track of the accumulated delay) while the connection establishment message passes downstream. The final flow specification is communicated to the target which may base its accept/reject decision on it. If a target accepts the connection, the flow specification is propagated back to the origin which can calculate an overall QOS for the entire connection for it. There is also a possibility to re-negotiate resource reservations if necessary.

3.4 Transport Layer

The core functions for multimedia communication as described in [Henckel, Stüttgen 1991] are already provided by the network layer. Thus, the transport layer of HeiTS is relatively light-weight. It makes the multicast and QOS functions visible to the transport users, hiding all details about intermediate nodes and how they contribute to the data transfer (i.e., how the routing tree is built, which QOS each individual hop has, etc.). In the HeiProjects, we design and implement HeiTP, the Heidelberg Transport Protocol [Delgrossi etc. 1992].

HeiTP adds to the multicast functions provided by the network layer the concept of complete and partial connections. A complete transport connection requires all targets to be available when the connection is established. A partial connection allows all entitled targets to join and leave the connection at their discretion. While complete connections are intended for individual conversation, partial connections support mass-based services such as TV distribution.

Data transport through networks – much unlike to data handling within a workstation – may always be subjected to errors. The transport layer, therefore, provides error detection and correction procedures. With increased network reliability, error functions for user data on a hop-by-hop basis become undesirable. To compensate for this if transport users require reliability, the receiving transport entity can perform error detection. Error correction can be achieved either by limited selective retransmission of messages (provided that throughput and delay guarantees are adjusted accordingly or not needed at all) or by forward error correction (provided that enough bandwidth for the required data redundancy is available) [Biersack 1991].

HeiTP also includes mechanisms for media scaling, i.e., adjusting the format of a media stream transmitted to the available bandwidth. This mechanism is used for networks which – even with the ST-II mechanisms – cannot dedicate bandwidth to certain users. The scaling procedure is implemented by having a monitor at each receiver keep track of the timeliness of incoming data. If data arrives too late, this is an indication of a system bottleneck. The protocol then triggers the source to reduce the amount of data sent, e.g., by lowering the video frame rate. The example is explained in more detail in [Delgrossi et al. 1993].

4 Multimedia Application Toolkit

Many distributed multimedia applications can be constructed from the same set of basic building blocks [Anderson, Chan 1991]. One such building block is the forwarding of multimedia data in real time as provided by stream handlers in general and by HeiTS in particular. In addition to data forwarding, distributed multimedia application entities require mechanisms to organize their cooperation. While these control functions usually require good performance and fast user feedback, they have no sharp deadlines and are, hence, not time-critical. They are located in the NRTE and do not require real-time communication protocols.

HeiMAT, the Heidelberg Multimedia Application Toolkit, is the subproject concerned with providing control functions for distributed multimedia applications. HeiMAT encompasses control primitives which complement the local multimedia functions and make them usable in a distributed environment. In [Käppner, Hehmann 1992] a list of design principles for HeiMAT is given. This list includes the following items:

- The toolkit functions need to support a diverse set of applications ranging from simple demo applications to full-fledged professional multimedia production systems.
- Whenever multimedia is involved, streaming serves a an illustrative paradigm. As in the local case (see Section 2.1), streaming should also be used as an abstraction for the distributed environment.
- Multimedia sources and sinks today use a variety of data formats. To, nevertheless, be able to connect them automatic data format conversion through filters is useful.

How HeiMAT works can either be specified by the user, the application or by the toolkit itself. For the first case, HeiMAT needs to provide a set of widgets to let the users specify settings they desire.

4.1 Architectural Approaches to a Multimedia Toolkit

Several approaches can, in principle, be taken to realize multimedia applications in a distributed system using the HeiMAT functions:

- HeiMAT-based modules can follow the client/server approach ("true distribution"). This would imply that every multimedia application is written in a way that takes distribution into account. This is shown in Figure 4.
- HeiMAT-based modules can follow the network transparency approach as made famous by the X window system ("invisible distribution"). In this case, multimedia applications are mainly unaware of being used in a network environment. This is shown in Figure 5.

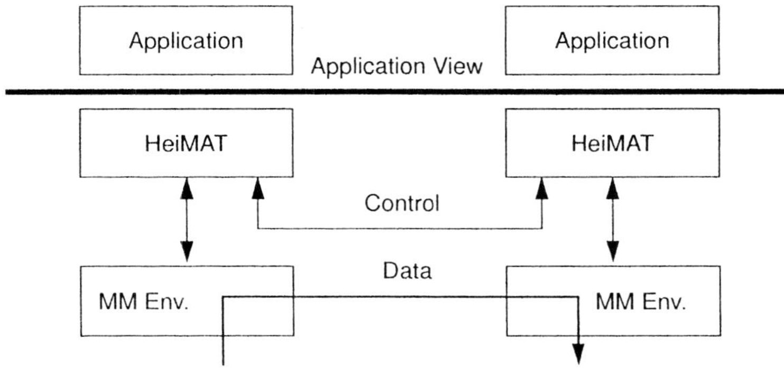

Figure 4: Distribution visible to application programmers (client/server)

Both approaches can be combined. In particular, a client/server system may use an I/O server such as X as its I/O abstraction. It may, however, not always use the networking functions of such a server.

Each approach has its justification: The client/server approach may lead to better performance and system response as it is possible to distinguish between local and remote execution of functions. For example, a stream stop operation could be performed locally, immediately freezing a video image on the screen. In the network-transparent case the stop function would always be sent to a remote application which may cause the video not to stop before one round-trip time.

On the other hand, with the network-transparent approach the application writer does not need to consider distribution when programming. One can come up with a solution similar to X to provide a universal I/O abstraction for multimedia. Unlike to X, however, data and control would follow different paths through the system. This is illustrated in Figure 5 where we see that each HeiMAT entity as part of an "AV server" for audio and video I/O communicates with the multimedia environment on its local machine to affect the flow of local multimedia streams.

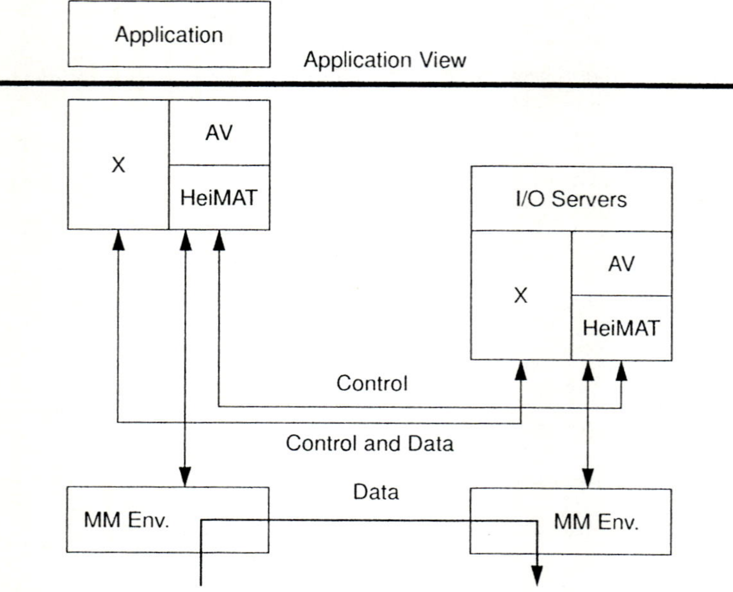

Figure 5: Distribution invisible to application programmers (network-transparent).

4.2 Main Function of a Multimedia Toolkit

The main function of a multimedia toolkit is to control the connection of audiovisual sources and sinks in a distributed environment. The transport system provides multicast connections from one origin to several targets and manages each connection for itself. Distributed multimedia applications often involve more than one source and, hence, more than one connection, often between more than two communication parties. The connections to be managed together either originate from the same node or from different nodes: If the audio and video of a movie are sent across different connections (e.g., because the dubbed soundtrack is not stored together with the images) both connections may come from the same node. In a phone conversation, one connection originates at each endpoint.

As multimedia transport connections are established in the direction from source to sink(s), the transport users have to exchange information on when to initiate a connection establishment or when to expect an incoming connection request. For example, to establish a phone call the caller has to inform its peer to initiate a backward connection. In this information phase, target and worst-case values for QOS parameters are communicated. This allows to avoid that, e.g., delays for individual connections are too far apart. Finally, the coordinated connection management can deal with situations where not all of the required connections are established, e.g., because the requested QOS is not available.

Synchronization of data arriving on different connections is an important issue. The synchronization itself is performed by the corresponding functions in the SMS, but it is the task of higher-level control functions to determine the correct settings of logical time systems to which the data shall be synchronized (see also [Steinmetz 1990]).

5 Elementary Multimedia Applications

The HeiProjects use a set of simple multimedia applications to test the function of the underlying modules. It happens that these demo applications also form the basic building blocks of more complicated applications as we discuss them in the following section.

5.1 Video Distribution

Television is one of the traditional media services. Therefore, it is obvious that such a broadcast-like distribution service qualifies as a future teleservice of distributed multimedia systems. Interaction between the sending and receiving peers in this distribution service is minimal. Receivers issue their request to get provided with a particular audio or video program.

To provide value-add service, audio and video programs can be distributed on demand. To utilize multicast functions and to reduce bandwidth requirements, it is common to cluster program requests. For example, the top 10 videos may only be available every 15 minutes. Users requesting such a video have to wait until the next start time.

Within the HeiProjects, HeiDI (the Heidelberg Video Distribution) performs the distribution of digital videos. The project is ongoing and results will be presented in a future paper.

5.2 Audiovisual Conferencing

Multi-party audio and video conferencing is another standard application for distributed multimedia systems, taking over and extending traditional telephone functions. Unlike to the multimedia distribution service, participation in the conferencing service is more balanced among the users. However, different degrees of balancing are possible. For teaching applications, e.g., it may be common that the flow of tutorial material is only rarely interrupted by questions of individual students.

Within the HeiProjects, an application called HeiPhone establishes multi-party audiovisual conferences among a group of users. The project is ongoing and results will be presented in a future paper.

6 Distributed Multimedia Teleservices

It should be obvious that one cannot provide a complete list of multimedia applications to be built on top of the infrastructural services described in the previous sections.

Some distributed multimedia applications qualify as multimedia teleservices for a large user community. The following subsections provide examples of how such services may look like.

6.1 Multimedia Kiosks

A multimedia kiosk is an information system that displays visual and acoustic data. The main application of kiosks is in public areas, e.g., as town, airport, or conference center information booths where easy access to information and easy-to-comprehend explanations – often in a multi-lingual way – are a key requirement.

Kiosks typically provides very simple and easy-to-use means for user input. Today's common kiosk input device is a touchscreen. In the future, speech recognition systems can become an important element of kiosk interfaces.

There is no single common way to implement multimedia kiosks. Yet, the kiosk paradigm can be realized through a generic kiosk framework. This program is then instantiated for the particular application.

6.2 Multimedia Mail

A multimedia mail application extends conventional electronic mail services like X.400 by the means to asynchronously exchange documents containing all kinds of media in arbitrary mixtures.[2] Mail documents do not contain hypermedia structures and are relatively short as far as their presentation is concerned – usually a few lines of text, a few seconds of video. Yet, even a few seconds of video can easily add up to several megabytes of data.

To participate in a mail service requires the ability to write and read notes and to distribute them. For writing and reading the same tool, an editor, can be used – e.g., an ODA [ISO 1989] editor. This editor will deal with text, graphics, and images. It has to be extended for the editing of audio and video, too. Among the functions needed for this purpose are stream editing (the rearrangement of recorded stream portions) and value editing (the modification of audio samples and video frames). Synthetic synchronization, to bring originally independent streams into some new temporal relationship (e.g., "start this audio piece ten seconds after that video portion"), is also a new editing function.

The distribution of documents in existing mail services follows a forward-and-store principle: Data is kept on the receiver's node. The large volume of mail containing audio and video may make this approach infeasible. Depending on storage constraints, the multimedia mail service leaves the mail message on the sending node (where it is stored already) or in a central archive and transmits it in real-time when the receiver wants to access it. Hence, for remote mail the multimedia mail application either uses the traditional transport service or HeiTS.

---

2. Experiments have shown, however, that only a few mail messages will contain both time-dependent and traditional media; often people either write or record their message, but not both [Hopper 1991].

The end-to-end delivery guarantees of HeiTS may make the real-time transfer also attractive if deterministic mail delivery is desired (as for registered letters), even if the data is stored on the receiver's node and not displayed immediately.

6.3 Multimedia Collaboration

Collaboration support can be provided in two ways: either through system software which makes existing applications sharable or through new applications which are "aware" of interfacing to several users. The first approach has the advantage of being able to run old applications in a collaborative fashion. The second approach requires new applications to be written, but may result in advanced functions as collaboration support is custom-made for the specific application.

Joint working is accomplished by workspaces accessible by several users at the same time. These workspaces can, e.g., include a sketchpad or a multimedia document editor. Each of them follows a different collaboration paradigm. In the sketchpad, one background image is displayed and each collaborator can draw sketches on this background image. The image can, e.g., be an engineering draft, an architectural plan, or a fashion design. It could also be a text that shall be annotated or corrected or a form that has to be filled out. Each user sees the sketches of all other users; the sketches are distinguished by different colors (corresponding to the icon colors of the communication windows). Sketches can be edited, combined, stored, etc.

For document editing, the background approach does not work: Editing modifies the original content of the document. Users can make their own modifications and then explicitly transmit their changes to all other participants. As no common background for reference exists, we find this less irritating than making each single editing function (potentially each keystroke including typing errors and their correction) immediately visible to all collaborators. Even in the process of joint editing, each author requires some privacy for the creative process of actually writing a document portion.

Unlike to the sketchpad, in joint editing each participant can have a different view on the document and individually browse through it. The editing process obviously needs to be coordinated, e.g., to avoid that one author has just modified a document portion only to find it deleted by someone else when he commits his new version. All traditional schemes of database locking, in principle, apply. One attractive solution is to enable authors to lock document portions, these portions are then highlighted in the author's color in each view of the document, and cannot be changed by any other author unless they are released. An alternative is to always build documents out of separate parts, each lockable.

The format of documents and the function set of the editor are arbitrary. One can use any existing editor and extend it by collaboration functions. Not starting to write a new editor from scratch ensures that design and development concentrates on the new collaboration aspects and is not sidetracked. The same applies to the graphic primitives of the sketchpad.

A joint working service usually is combined with a multimedia conferencing service as audiovisual communication is an ideal means for coordinating collaboration.

Acknowledgments

The HeiProjects are a group effort. Many discussions with my fellow project members have influenced this paper. I would like to express my gratitude to all members of the former AIX and OS/2 project members who have made the transition from their individual work items to a common project framework. That the HeiProjects are now an effort that spans both platforms is due to the dedication and encouragement of people from both sides. We could not have done it without you!

References

Anderson, D., Chan, P. (1991): Toolkit Support for Multiuser Audio/Video Applications. Second International Workshop for Network and Operating System Support for Digital Audio and Video, Heidelberg, Lecture Notes in Computer Science, Springer, Heidelberg, November 1991.

Anderson, D., Govindan, R., Homsy, G. (1991): Abstractions for Continuous Media in a Network Window System. International Conference on Multimedia Information Systems, Singapore, January 1991.

Anderson, D., Homsy, G. (1991): A Continuous-Media I/O Server and Its Synchronization Mechanism. IEEE Computer, Vol. 24, No. 10, October 1991.

Anderson, D., Tzou, S.-Y., Wahbe, R., Govindan, R., Andrews, M. (1990): Support for Continuous-Media in the DASH System. International Conference on Distributed Computing Systems, Paris, 1990.

Biersack, E. (1991): A Performance Study of Forward Error Correction in ATM Networks. Second International Workshop for Network and Operating System Support for Digital Audio and Video, Heidelberg, Lecture Notes in Computer Science, Springer, Heidelberg, November 1991.

Bocke, P., Armbruster, H. (1991): Broadband Services – An Overview. Telecommunications. Vol. 25, No. 12, December 1991.

Davies, N.A., Nicol, J.R. (1991): Technological Perspective on Multimedia Computing. Computer Communications, Vol. 14, No. 5, June 1991.

Delgrossi, L., Halstrick, C., Herrtwich, R.G., Stüttgen, H.J. (1992): HeiTP – A Transport Protocol for ST-II. Globecom '92, Orlando, December 1992.

Delgrossi, L., Halstrick, C., Hehmann, D., Herrtwich, R.G., Krone, O., Sandvoss, J., Vogt, C.: Media Scaling for Audiovisual Communication with the Heidelberg Transport System, ACM Multimedia 93, Anaheim, August 1993.

Ferrari, D. (1991): Design and Applications of a Delay Jitter Control Scheme for Packet-Switching Internetworks. Second International Workshop for Network and Operating System Support for Digital Audio and Video, Heidelberg, Lecture Notes in Computer Science, Springer, Heidelberg, November 1991.

Fox, E.A. (1991a): Standards and the Emergence of Digital Multimedia Systems. Communications of the ACM, Vol. 34, No. 4, April 1991.

Fox, E.A. (1991b): Advances in Interactive Digital Multimedia Systems. IEEE Computer, Vol. 24, No. 10, October 1991.

Hanko, J.G., Kuerner, E.G., Northcutt, J.D., Wall, G.A. (1991): Workstation Support for Time-Critical Applications. Second International Workshop for Network and Operating System Support for Digital Audio and Video, Heidelberg, Lecture Notes in Computer Science, Springer, Heidelberg, November 1991.

Hehmann, D., Herrtwich, R.G., Steinmetz, R. (1991a): Creating HeiTS: Objectives of the Heidelberg High-Speed Transport System. Technical Report, IBM European Networking Center, Heidelberg, October 1991.

Hehmann, D., Köhler, B., Luttenberger, N., Mackert, L., Schulz, W., Stüttgen, H. (1991b): Implementation Experience with a Communication Subsystem Prototype for B-ISDN. Third Conference on High-Speed Networking, IFIP, Berlin, March 1991.

Hehmann, D., Salmony, M., Stüttgen, H. (1989): Transport Services for Multimedia Applications. IFIP Workshop on Protocols for High-Speed Networks, 1989.

Henckel, L., Stüttgen, H. (1991): Transportdienste in Breitbandnetzen. Kommunikation in verteilten Systemen, Mannheim, Informatik-Fachberichte, Springer, Heidelberg, February 1991.

Herrtwich, R.G. (1991a): The Role of Performance, Scheduling, and Resource Reservation in Multimedia Systems. Operating Systems of the 90s and Beyond. Dagstuhl Workshop, Lecture Notes in Computer Science, Springer, Heidelberg, 1991.

Herrtwich, R.G. (1991b): Time Capsules – An Abstraction for Access to Continuous-Media Data. Journal of Real-Time Systems, Vol. 3, No. 4, December 1991.

Herrtwich, R.G., Steinmetz, R. (1991): Towards Integrated Multimedia Systems – Why and How?. GI-Jahrestagung, Darmstadt, Informatik-Fachbericht, Springer-Verlag, Heidelberg, October 1991 (also Technical Report 43.9101, IBM European Networking Center, Heidelberg).

Herrtwich, R.G. (1992): An Architecture for Multimedia Data Stream Handling and Its Implication for Multimedia Transport Service Interfaces. Third IEEE Workshop on Future Trends of Distributed Computing Systems, Taipei, April 1992.

Hopper., A. (1991): Personal Communication, November 1991 (See also: Herrtwich, R.G. (Ed.): Summary of the Second International Workshop on Network and Operating System Support for Digital Audio and Video, ACM Computer Communication Review, Vol. 22, No. 2, April 1992).

IBM (1991): Ultimedia Digest. IBM Corporation, 1991.

IBM (1992): Multimedia Presentation Manager/2, Programming Reference. IBM Corporation, 1992.

ISO (1989): Office Document Architecture and Interchange Format. International Standard 8613, International Organization for Standardization, Geneva, 1989.

Käppner, T., Hehmann, D. (1992): Objectives of HeiMAT – The Heidelberg Multimedia Application Toolkit. Third International Workshop on Network and Operating System Support for Digital Audio and Video, San Diego, November 1992.

Krueger, M.W. (1991): Artificial Reality II. Addison-Wesley, Reading, 1991.

Mc Kellar, B.: Buffer Management in Communication Systems. Technical Report, IBM European Networking Center, Heidelberg, 1993.

Nagarajan, R., Vogt, C. (1992): Guaranteed-Performance Transport of Multimedia Traffic over the Token Ring. Technical Report 43.9201, IBM European Networking Center, Heidelberg, January 1992.

Rangan, V., Vin, H.M. (1991): Designing File Systems for Digital Audio and Video. Thirteenth ACM Symposium on Operating Systems Principles, Pacific Grove, ACM Operating Systems Review, Vol. 25, No.5, October 1991.

Rheingold, H. (1991): Virtual Reality. Summit Books, New York, 1991.

Steinmetz, R. (1990): Synchronization Properties in Multimedia Systems. IEEE Journal on Selected Areas in Communication, Vol. 8, No. 3, April 1990.

Steinmetz, R., Schmutz, H., Schöner, B., Wasmund, M. (1990): Generic Support for Distributed Multimedia Applications. ICC '90, IEEE, Atlanta, April 1990 (also Technical Report 43.8910, IBM European Networking Center, Heidelberg).

Topolcic, C. (Ed., 1990): Experimental Internet Stream Protocol, Version 2 (ST-II). Internet Request for Comments 1190, Network Working Group, October 1990.

Vogt, C., Herrtwich, R.G., Nagarajan, R. (1992): HeiRAT – The Heidelberg Resource and Administration Technique – Design Philosophy and Goals. Technical Report, IBM European Networking Center, Heidelberg, July 1992.

X/Open (1988): X/Open Portability Guide: Networking Services. X/Open Company, Ltd., Prentice-Hall, Englewood Cliffs, 1988.

Database Management for Multimedia Applications

Klaus Meyer-Wegener
Technical University of Dresden, Faculty of Computer Science, Institute of Software Engineering II, 01062 Dresden, Germany

Abstract

In multimedia computer systems, the data objects created, stored, manipulated, and presented differ from the data objects used in other systems. Digitized images, sound, and video ask for new methods in data management. In this paper, the task of data management for multimedia applications is defined and clearly distinguished from other tasks like editing and complex analysis. Next, the main services are identified and described, i.e. data abstraction, representation of relationships, and search. This leads to a particular interface of multimedia database management systems that is illustrated using the Abstract Data Type IMAGE and the relational data model. The implementation of such an interface is on its way, but some issues are still open and need further research. Content-oriented search is the most important one. The paper concludes with an outlook on other research problems in the field.

1 Introduction: What Is Multimedia?

The starting point for the development of multimedia computer systems is the availability of hardware which allows to *capture* and *present* information in a variety of media, e.g. text, image, and sound. The media can be used alternatively or even in parallel. This reduces the need to code information on input and thus makes it easier for non-skilled (or non-willing) users to enter data. On output, the means for presenting information can be chosen from a much richer set, and in some cases, the choice can be postponed until access time and then be left to the user.

However, the improvement of user interfaces, or the increase in information bandwidth between system and user, as it is sometimes characterized [Woel85a], is only one effect of multimedia. There is also *more information* held in the system: If a photograph is captured and later presented, more information is given to the users than could ever by use of formatted (coded) data. This information, of course, is not easy to process mechanically, but it can be stored and retrieved. And this means that there is a data management task in the design and implementation of multimedia systems.

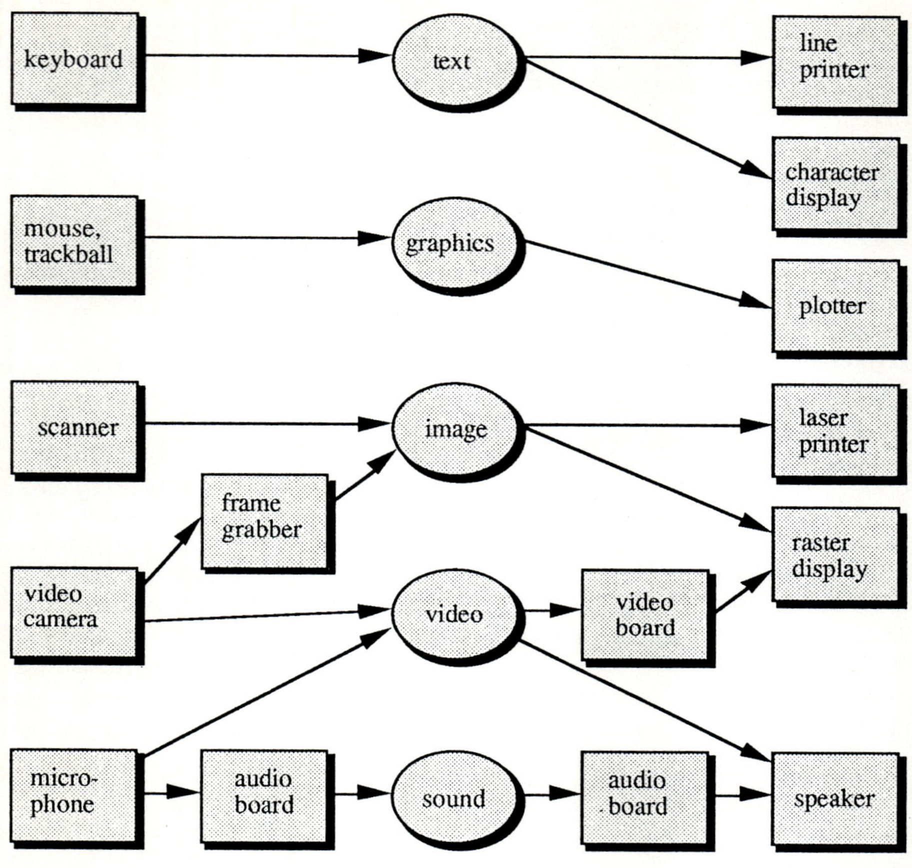

Fig. 1. Relationship of input/output devices and media data

2 DBMS Technology and Multimedia

The new input devices (scanners, cameras, sound boards, etc.) produce new types of data objects. Due to their size, they must often be placed on special kinds of storage devices , e.g. on optical storage or even on VCR's. Their main purpose is to be available for rendering on certain output devices (raster displays, sound boards, video boards). However, to be fed into those output devices, they must have a specific format required by the device, and in many cases, the original format of capture needs to be modified and converted. Sometimes media data objects are not obtained from capture but are computed from other data, e.g. from 3D models or measurement data (visualization, animation). In that case, the data format is usually chosen to match the output devices that are available. Fig. 1 shows the different types of data objects in between the input and output devices.

Until now, experimental systems use only small sets of those media data objects. As more and more applications are extended with multimedia facilities, the volume of the data will grow significantly, and their management will reach a new quality. It will not be possible to remember all the objects by their names, hence search based on different criteria should be possible. Also, the environment (software and hardware configurations) will change while the data remain valid, so that some kind of openness and application neutrality should be provided. This poses new challenges on the data management which can no longer be achieved in an ad-hoc manner. The question is whether DBMS technology can be helpful in accomplishing the task. DBMS's are powerful, yet expensive software packages. Mainly, they offer the following services:

- data independence (data abstraction)
- application neutrality (openness)
- versatile query language (unanticipated data access)
- multi-user operation (concurrency control)
- fault tolerance (transactions, recovery)
- access control (security)

In this paper, it is suggested that these services can be extended to apply to multimedia data as well, and that the development of multimedia applications can benefit from the availability of such a DBMS.

3 DBMS as Part of a Multimedia System

In contrast to other approaches, it is intended here to develop a DBMS that serves just as a base tool for multimedia system development, not as a stand-alone system that is used side-by-side with others. Hence, the services are primarily offered to the multimedia application programmer, not to the end-user. The underlying hypothesis is that a DBMS should be responsible for the *storage* and *retrieval* of multimedia data objects, not more and not less. *Not more* means that complex processing, e.g. of images, is not the task of DBMS. Neither is the lengthy process of editing. Instead, analysis programs and editors should be able to obtain their data from the database and to later file their results in the database if they wish. *Not less* means that a file system or a (relational) DBMS with just "binary large objects" (BLOBs) falls short of the quality of data management already available for formatted data, particularly with respect to data independence. Similarly, an "atomized" storage where words of a text or pixels of an image are managed as separate entities (e.g. in tuples of a relation), fails to meet the needs of most applications that want to treat the data objects as a whole.

4 Benefits for Multimedia Systems from DBMS Technology

Even when restricting the task of a DBMS to storage and retrieval, some interesting problems have to be solved [Masu87a]. A *data model* for multimedia data must be developed that allows to store and retrieve them without being forced to go down to the bits and bytes of data representation. Data management should isolate the user (i.e. the programmer) from the details of storage device management and from the details of the storage formats used. Then both may be changed without affecting the applications.

As mentioned before, the storage of multimedia data objects requires the use of special storage devices (optical disks, VCR's) that have other characteristics than the standard magnetic disks [Laub86a]. If the applications have to take these characteristics into account, they are tied to the device used for a specific object. Moving that data object to another device or replacing the device with a more advanced one then requires program modifications. The lesson learned in data management that led to the development of today's DBMS for formatted data is that *device independence* should be achieved in the applications, so that reorganization of device allocation will leave the programs as they are.

Multimedia data objects also come in a rich variety of data formats (data structures). For instance, images can be coded in GIF, TIFF, PBM, FBM, Pixmap, and many other formats. Which format is most appropriate depends on the application environment and the I/O devices at hand. Since a multimedia DBMS is supposed to support many applications, it will have to host many different formats, too. In particular, a certain media object, e.g. an image, can be shared by different applications that would like to see it in their respective formats. It is the task of the multimedia DBMS to provide *format independence* to the applications, i.e. to supply each the format it needs while hiding the internal storage format actually used. So if 80 % of the applications need an image in GIF, the internal format could be GIF, too, and a conversion is performed for the remaining 20 %. However, if the application profile changes and now 80 % need the same image in PBM format, the internal format can be switched to PBM without any application program being affected. Format independence also covers the usage of two different internal formats for the same image, if the applications are split fifty-to-fifty. Since this is completely under control of the DBMS, consistent update of the two copies is guaranteed.

Single-medium data objects are usually not on their own, but are related with other media objects and with formatted data. There are at least three types of *relationships* that a multimedia DBMS should be able to represent and to use for retrieval:

- *Object-attribute relationship:* Objects (or entities) like ships, cars, persons, etc. can also be described by photos, graphics, and sound recordings. Thus a media object shows a property of the object represented in the system.
- *Aggregate-component relationship:* Multimedia data objects, mostly documents, are composed of a number of single-medium data objects. The components are not just attributes, but entities in their own right. There may be additional rela-

tionships among the components, of which the synchronization (e.g. show text and graphic together) is the most important [Stei89a].

– *Substitution relationship:* The same information can often be represented in different media, e.g. as a table (formatted) or as a graph. Automatic translation is possible in some cases, but in others it is not (sound to text). Hence, it can be necessary to store both representations to be able to cope with different workstation configurations and user preferences. In that case, a link should be maintained between the two to allow for substitution. This means the DBMS can switch to the alternative representation when required, and it can warn the users when just one of the equivalent objects is updated.

Finally, *search* for media data objects is the task of the DBMS. It cannot be done efficiently by the applications themselves. If the media objects to be retrieved can be identified with the help of associated formatted data, standard DBMS techniques can be used. If the media objects themselves have to be inspected, pattern matching can be performed. Data structures and algorithms have been developed to increase its efficiency significantly (e.g. signature files for text [Falo85a] and iconic indexing for images [Chan87a]). Neither of the two covers what is usually called *content addressability* of media data objects: Many things represented in an image will not be coded as formatted data ("storm", "foggy night"), and it can be very hard to find the right pattern to retrieve only relevant images. There are no pat solutions at hand for this; some preliminary results are given in [Meye91a].

Device independence, format independence, representation of relationships, and content search must all be reflected in the data model. The modelling concepts must be complemented with a set of operations that store, manipulate, and retrieve the data in a consistent way. Finding a basic and wisely restricted set of DBMS functions that support a variety of application programs seems to be the most important design issue for a multimedia database system.

Table 1. Important Characteristics of Media Data Objects

Medium	*Elements*	*Organization*	*Typical ranges of sizes*	*Time-dependency?*	*Human sense*
Text	Characters	Sequence	1 K - 1 M	No	Visual and auditory
Graphics	Lines, areas	Set	1 K - 10 M	No	Visual
Raster image	Pixels	Matrix	1 - 100 M	No	Visual
Sound	Amplitude values	Sequence	1 - 600 M	Yes	Auditory
Video (moving image)	Raster images or graphics	Sequence	1 - 100 G	Yes	Visual

5 Development of a Multimedia DBMS

The task of a multimedia DBMS is to manage large volumes of multimedia data, such that users can store and retrieve them without referring to devices and formats. To accomplish this, the data objects to be stored must be investigated carefully. Table 1 shows the main characteristics of the media data objects; a more detailed description can be found in [Lock88a, Meye92a], for instance.

5.1 Data Model

It is widely accepted that the media data objects should be managed as instances of Abstract Data Types. This makes it easy to guarantee device and format independence and also provides a framework to implement search facilities. However, it does not help in composing higher-level multimedia data objects, i.e. documents, out of the media data objects. Nor does it provide any means to represent other kinds of relationships. To do this, an embedding of the Abstract Data Types in a generic data model is needed.

Many scientists claim that the data model of a multimedia DBMS can only be object-oriented [Woel86a, Woel87a, Masu87a]. Unfortunately, object-oriented DBMS are still subject to lively development, and the numerous proposals and prototypes differ in many aspects [Atki89a]. It is far from clear today which of the proposals will finally prevail. So building multimedia management on top of one of the systems will yield only a specific solution with little implications for the other environments. Even worse, the proposals for multimedia DBMS usually define their own object-oriented data model and thus add to the variety.

On the other side, many people with a background in relational and extensible DBMS claim that starting from scratch is not necessary [Ston90a]. It has been shown in many research projects since 1980 that relational systems can be extended to support Abstract Data Types among other things [Hask82a, Ong84a]. At the same time, they offer the benefits of well-tested, optimized, standardized, and established systems.

The controversy is still in a very heated phase. Instead of favoring one of the opposing parties, it is also possible to define the Abstract Data Types independently of the data model. Then they can later be integrated into a standard relational data model as domains and into an object-oriented data model as classes or types. To illustrate the embedding in the following sections, the extended relational model will be used. The reason is that most readers will be familar with the relational model, so that lengthy explanations are not required. However, this does not mean that object-orientation is irrelevant for multimedia data; very interesting research is done in this area, e.g. [Klas90a, Klas92a].

5.2 The Data Type IMAGE as an Example

Raster images will be used as an example to demonstrate the definition of an Abstract Data Type for media data objects. The definition of data types and operators for the other media can be done in a similar way and will not be presented here.

An IMAGE value is more than just a matrix of pixels. It contains some other information such as height, width, pixel depth, color definition, colormap, etc. These registration data are mandatory, since they are needed to render the image properly, and hence are included in the IMAGE value. This is sketched in Fig. 2.

As in any Abstract Data Type, the components are only accessible through functions. This is to hide the internal strorage structures and formats used to represent them and thus fulfills the requirement to make the programs device independent and format independent. The function create_image assembles an IMAGE value from the contents of program variables and constants. It checks the parameter values for consistency and maps them to whatever internal format used for the images. Please note that the encoding parameter indicates only how the input in pixelmatrix and colormap has to be interpreted, and does not imply any preference for the internal format.

```
create_image    (height : INTEGER,
                width : INTEGER,
                depth : INTEGER,
                aspect_ratio : REAL,
                encoding : CODE,
                colormap_length : INTEGER,
                colormap_depth : INTEGER,
                colormap : ARRAY [2:*, 1:*] OF INTEGER,
                pixelmatrix : ARRAY [1:*] OF BIT
                ) : IMAGE;
```

Other create functions can be defined that use specific image formats as input parameters and thus reduce the number of parameters significantly. Access to components of an IMAGE value is performed with the help of functions like:

```
height (i : IMAGE) : INTEGER;
width (i : IMAGE) : INTEGER;
```

Again, specific data structures used in some application environments (e.g. Ximage) can be filled with an IMAGE value in a single function call. In an interactive environment, loading data structures is of no use; one would like to display an image on a monitor or in a separate window of the screen:

```
display (i : IMAGE; d : DEVICE) : BOOLEAN;
```

The return value of this function indicates whether the display operation was successful or not. Modifying IMAGE values must also be done through functions that guarantee consistent update of raw data and registration data. Examples are:

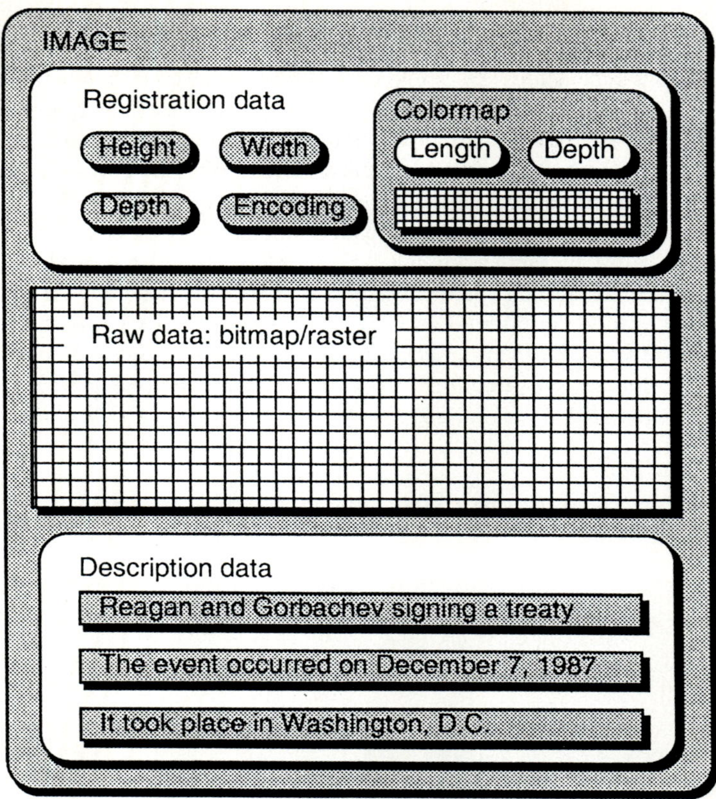

Fig. 2. Conceptual view of an instance or value of the Abstract Data Type IMAGE

```
replace_colormap
    (i : IMAGE,
    encoding : CODE,
    colormap_length : INTEGER,
    colormap_depth : INTEGER,
    colormap : ARRAY [2:*, 1:*] OF INTEGER
    ) : IMAGE;
replace_pixelvalue
    (i : IMAGE,
    x, y : INTEGER,
    pixelvalue : ARRAY [1:*] OF BIT
    ) : IMAGE;
```

This list of examples is anything but complete. We are convinced that many applications will add specific functions to derive other data from an `IMAGE` value or to perform complex updates in a single call. The DBMS must be flexible enough to allow for the definition of those functions. After some experience, a sufficiently large library will be available to new users.

Next, a proper embedding of the ADT's into a data model is needed to allow for the representation of relationships among the data objects and to get the power of a query language for access. In the relational model, the ADT's defined for media data objects (like the `IMAGE` shown above) can be used as domains. If a relational DBMS offers a facility to define new domains, the embedding can be done in a straight-forward manner. University Ingres [Ong84a] and its successor Postgres [Ston86a] offer such a facility, although it is not perfecly suited to multimedia data. In the following we shall assume that such a facility exists.

Since `IMAGE` is a domain, an image is supposed to be handled as an attribute value of some object or entity (a ship or an aircraft, for instance). Usually it is an attribute of the object shown on the picture. Also, more than one attributes of type `IMAGE` can be defined for a relation. Typical examples are:

```
Employee     (EmpNo              INTEGER,
              ....
              Portrait           IMAGE)

Inmate       (InmNo              INTEGER,
              ....
              FrontView          IMAGE,
              SideView           IMAGE,
              FingerPrints       IMAGE)

Car          (Manufacturer       STRING,
              YearBuilt          INTEGER,
              ....
              Photo              IMAGE,
              EngineSound        SOUND)
```

This kind of schema easily models the object-attribute relationship demanded in Sect. 4. More complex database schemas can be defined to model other types of relationships [Meye92a].

To give an impression of the access to a relational database that holds media objects, an integration of the ADT operators with a query language will be shown. SQL is taken as the query language, since it is in wide-spread use and has been standardized by ANSI and ISO [ANSI86a].

The example relation used in the queries is even simpler than the ones shown above; it consists of two attributes only:

```
AerialPhoto     (No      INTEGER,
                 Photo   IMAGE)
```

To store tuples in this relation, the normal SQL `INSERT` statement is used:

```
INSERT INTO AerialPhoto
VALUES (:number, create_image (512, 480, 8, ... ));
```

The leading colon distinguishes program variable names from relation names and attribute names. It is important that type checking can be done at compile time already. The first entry in the value clause must specify a value for the attribute No and must thus be of type INTEGER. Accordingly, the second entry must be of type IMAGE. Since the result type of the operation create_image is in fact IMAGE, the compiler accepts the function call.

An update operation that includes an IMAGE attribute must also use an operator which returns an IMAGE value. For instance:

```
UPDATE AerialPhoto
SET Photo = replace_colormap (Photo, RGB, 256, 24, :cm)
WHERE No = 1234;
```

To select particular images from the database, the usual SQL expressions can be used to identify the tuples. However, the typical comparison of attribute values and constants is only allowed for the standard data types. So again the operators must be used to extract components that have INTEGER or BIT values, before a comparison can be performed:

```
SELECT height (Photo), width (Photo)
INTO :h, :w
FROM AerialPhoto
WHERE encoding (Photo) = RGB_COLORMAP
AND depth (Photo) = 8;
```

The example also shows how an IMAGE value can be retrieved from the database. Since its format must be hidden, it cannot be assigned directly to a program variable as a whole. Operators are used to select components with basic data types or structured data types like arrays that can be assigned to program variables. Given a specific environment, additional operators can be defined to fill a complex record structure in a single call (e.g. Ximage).

While the relationships among the data objects support a navigational access, there is also a need to search in a descriptive way, i.e. to provide properties or patterns of the data objects wanted and have the DBMS find the set of matching objects. Many different ways of approaching this problem of "content addressability" are known; they must be classified and evaluated.

5.3 Search

To search a large set of multimedia data objects is a prime task for a multimedia DBMS. In what has been discussed so far, it can be done using the standard formatted attributes associated with the media objects, or using result values of operators. This is easily implemented with standard database search techniques (e.g. indexing), but it will not suffice to answer all questions. Certain phenomena shown on images will hardly be represented by attributes or relations (as are ships, persons, horses, cars), e.g. "storm," "fog," "night," etc. So the media object itself must be used in the qualification.

Pattern matching is a technique that can do just that. Full-text retrieval is an example. However, little meaning is involved in the comparison of the pattern and the raw data. In the case of image and sound, it can be very hard to find the right pattern. If you are looking for photos of a snowstorm, you must specify something like "lots of white pixels," which does not necessarily match only snowstorms, nor does it match all snowstorm images.

What is desirable lies somewhat in between: It does take the media object itself into account, but it compares on a more semantical level. For instance, one would like to find:

- mugshots on the basis of witnesses' reports: beady eyes, long nose, etc.
- aerial photos that show an airport (a river, an industry plant, ...)
- press photos of Bush and Gorbachev signing a treaty
- text passages on the subject of urban traffic
- recordings of interviews on speed limits.

It is obvious that questions like these cannot easily be mapped to pattern matching. Run-time analysis of a media object would be appropriate (e.g. run a specific image analysis to find airports), but is simply not possible with today's technology. Text understanding and speech recognition only work in restricted domains and are still pretty costly. The only way out is to do the analysis off-line and store the results together with the media objects.

As a consequence, the task of generating the content descriptions is delegated to the users of the DBMS (remember they are programmers). They may run complex image analysis and text understanding software to do so, or may just as well decide to enter the descriptions manually. As of today, the latter will still produce the better descriptions, but it can be too time-consuming in some situations. However, authors have been living with the obligation to provide the keywords along with their texts for some time now. The task of the DBMS then is to store the descriptions and to use them in search for the multimedia objects.

The next question is how these content descriptions of media data objects should look like. Formatted data have already been ruled out because of their lack of expressiveness, although they could be searched efficiently. At least four other types of descriptions could be considered:

- keywords
- knowledge representation
- natural-language text
- restricted text (captions).

Keywords have been used in libraries and in information retrieval systems for a long time. Elaborated techniques are available to perform search on the basis of keyword descriptors [Salt83a]. The expressiveness however is still to weak to describe the contents of pictures, sound recordings, and video. Interdependencies, complex sequences of actions, and causal connections can hardly be represented. Knowledge representation techniques on the other hand are rich enough to model them, and they also lend themselves to efficient search. The only problem with them is that they are rather hard to understand. Unskilled users are not able to work with them directly;

they need a "knowledge engineer" who maps their expertise onto knowledge representation structures.

Natural-language text has just the opposite characteristics: It is easy to generate, but it is hard to search. Expressiveness is as good as with knowledge representation, if not better. However, text descriptions are themselves unformatted and thus not very helpful in conducting search. Full-text search is the only appropriate method, and it still bears the problems of pattern matching. Actually, the scope of content addressability has only been shifted from an arbitrary medium to the single medium "text," but that is no solution.

As a compromise, restricted text, in particular captions (noun phrases), could be used. They are almost as easy to write as free text, but at the same time can be processed and turned into knowledge representations used internally for search. This yields both easy input of descriptions, even by laymen, and efficient and well-defined search. It seems appropriate to look into this approach a little further and to enumerate the consequences [Lum90a].

5.4 Architecture

The media data types, their embedding into a data model, and the extension of the query language with the operators define the functionality of a multimedia DBMS. The next question is how such a DBMS could be implemented.

A software system of the size and complexity of a DBMS should be decomposed into modules. Traditionally, these modules are organized in layers as described for instance in [Härd83a]. However, performance is much more important when real-time requirements for audio and video data must be satisfied, so the layers must not cause a significant software overhead. Instead, the goal should be to minimize the number of copying and mapping operations, even if this forces compromises with respect to data independence.

The facilities that support content search must also be added to the conventional DBMS architecture. This includes a parser for the captions, a matcher for stored descriptions and queries, and a description manager that organizes large sets of content descriptions for efficient search. Standard database storage structures cannot be used for the descriptions, new ones must be developed. For some ideas in this respect see [Lum90a].

The task then is to move from well-established DBMS to new multimedia DBMS. Many concepts have been developed to achieve "extensible" DBMS, some of which are useful for the handling of multimedia data (e.g. an ADT definition facility) while others are not (access path definition based on total ordering). A thorough evaluation with respect to multimedia data management remains to be done.

Masunaga has developed a framework that helps to classify and compare the architectures defined in the research projects [Masu87a]. He assumes different database systems for the different media. They are integrated using an additional object-oriented database that refers to them. There is either a single (extensible) DBMS managing all these different databases ("single DBMS architecture"), a "primary" multimedia DBMS that calls the "secondary" media-specific DBMS as subroutines ("primary-secondary DBMS architecture"), or a collection of cooperating DBMS accessing each other via Remote Data Access ("federated DBMS architecture").

A very detailed proposal for a multimedia DBMS architecture is given in [Lock88a]. As in the primary-secondary architecture, media-specific data management systems are integrated into a single system, but they are supposed to be all based on a common object-oriented system. Only the video management system has its own storage system, since it must use a VCR instead of magnetic and optical disks. In addition to the media-specific systems, the architecture hosts a "mixed-object manager" and an "interrelationship manager." Their task is to provide the integration of single-media objects into multimedia objects (mostly documents) and the management of various types of relationships among the media objects, respectively.The user interacts with the system through a homogeneous interface that hides the media-specific data management systems. The functionality of this interface however is still an open issue.

6 Research Issues

The *extensibility mechanisms* proposed today in relational and in object-oriented systems must be tested and evaluated on multimedia data. Some of them work nicely for "complex number" and "box," but lead to a very awkward modelling when applied to images. Also, extensibility in some cases does not allow the inclusion of new storage devices such as a VCR.

The handling of *meta-data* deserves more attention. When working with multimedia data, the users often want to know about the source and quality of the data since it determines the information content. Also, the representation of structure and content is essential for an effective search.

The embedding into the data model usually provides a mechanism to define *relationships*. However, these relationships are not distinguished with respect to the special needs of multimedia data. More semantics could be added by defining, for instance, a synchronisation relationship. Update operations on the data must then respect the special semantics of these relationships.

The *implementation* of a DBMS that handles multimedia data in the way described is not fully understood. Some proposals include a federated architecture with media-specific management systems, while others envision a single system powerful enough for all media. Performance is a very important issue, since the time-dependent media (sound and video) are also the ones that produce extremely large data objects. This affects among others database buffer management.

Even if all this has been solved, the *design of the ADTs* for the multimedia data objects still remains a difficult job. A trade-off exists between the need for data independence and the flexible use of the data objects. Ideally, using a function to access the object should be as easy as de-referencing a pointer – at least syntactically.

While many problems of multimedia data management remain to be solved, the design and implementation of data-independent multimedia applications today can give room to numerous optimizations and preserves the investment in application development without being tied to current storage technology.

Acknowledgements

The author greatly appreciates the helpful comments of the anonymous referee.

References

ANSI86a ANSI, *The Database Language SQL,* Document ANSI X3.133, 1986.

Atki89a Atkinson, M., Bancilhon, F., DeWitt, D., Dittrich, K., Maier, D., and Zdonik, S., "The Object-Oriented Database System Manifesto," in *Proc. 1st Int. Conf. on Deductive and Object-Oriented Databases* (Kyoto, Japan, Dec. 1989), eds. W. Kim, J.-M. Nicolas, and S. Nishio, Elsevier Science Publishers, B.V., Amsterdam, 1989, pp. 40–57.

Chan87a Chang, S.-K., Shi, Q.-Y., and Yan, C.-W., "Iconic Indexing by 2-D Strings," *IEEE Trans. on Pattern Analysis and Machine Intelligence,* vol. PAMI-9, no. 3, May 1987, pp. 413–428.

Falo85a Faloutsos, C., "Access Methods for Text," *ACM Computing Surveys,* vol. 17, no. 1, March 1985, pp. 49–74.

Härd83a Härder, T., and Reuter, A., "Concepts for Implementing a Centralized Database Management System," in *Proc. Int. Computing Symposium 1983 on Application Systems Development* (ICS 83, Nürnberg), Teubner Verlag, Stuttgart 1983, pp. 28–59.

Hask82a Haskin, R., and Lorie, R., "On Extending the Functions of a Relational Database System," in *Proc. ACM SIGMOD Conf.* (June 1982), pp. 207–212.

Klas90a Klas, W., Neuhold, E.J., and Schrefl, M., "Using an Object-Oriented Approach to Model Multimedia Data," Report, GMD-IPSI, Darmstadt, Germany, May 1990, 28 pp.,published in *Computer Communications,* Special Issue on Multimedia Systems, vol. 13, no. 4, May 1990, pp.204–216.

Klas92a Klas, W., "Tailoring an Object-Oriented Database System to Integrate External Multimedia Devices," ICSI, Berkeley, CA, 1992?

Laub86a Laub, L., "The Evolution of Mass Storage," *Byte,* vol. 11, no. 5, May 1986, pp. 161–172.

Lock88a Lockemann, P.C., "Multimedia Databases: Paradigm, Architecture, Survey and Issues," report no. NPS52-88-047, Naval Postgraduate School, Monterey, CA, Sept. 1988.

Lum90a Lum, V.Y., and Meyer-Wegener, K., "An Architecture for a Multimedia Database Management System Supporting Content Search," in *Proc. Int. Conf. on Computing and Information* (ICCI '90, Niagara Falls, Canada, May 1990).

Masu87a Masunaga, Y., "Multimedia Databases: A Formal Framework," in *Proc. IEEE CS Office Automation Symp.* (Gaithersburg, MD, Apr. 1987), IEEE CS Press, order no. 770, Washington, 1987, pp. 36–45.

Meye91a Meyer-Wegener, K., *Multimedia-Datenbanken* (Multimedia Databases), B.G. Teubner, Leitfäden der angewandten Informatik, Stuttgart 1991 (in German).

Meye92a Meyer-Wegener, K., "Multimedia Databases: Integrated Storage and Retrieval of Text, Images, Sound and Video," Bericht Nr. 92/2 des Sonderforschungsbereichs 182 Multiprozessor- und Netzwerkkonfigurationen, Teilprojekt B4, Arbeitsberichte des IMMD, Universität Erlangen-Nürnberg, Bd. 25, Nr. 12, Erlangen, Nov. 1992 (in English).

Ong84a Ong, J., Fogg, D., and Stonebraker, M., "Implementation of Data Abstraction in the Relational Database System INGRES," *ACM SIGMOD Record,* vol. 14, no. 1, 1984, pp. 1–14.

Salt83a Salton, G., and McGill, M.J., *Introduction to Modern Information Retrieval,* McGraw-Hill, New York 1983.

Stei89a Steinmetz, R., "Synchronization Properties in Multimedia Systems," Technical Report No. 43.8906, IBM European Networking Center, Heidelberg, May 1989.

Ston86a Stonebraker, M., and Rowe, L.A., "The Design of POSTGRES," in *Proc. ACM SIGMOD '86* (Washington, May 1986), ed. C. Zaniolo, also *ACM SIGMOD Record,* vol. 15, no. 2, June 1986, pp. 208–214.

Ston90a Stonebraker, M., Rowe, L., Lindsay, B., Gray, J., Carey, M., Brodie, M., Bernstein, P., and Beech, D., "Third-Generation Database System Manifesto," *ACM SIGMOD Record,* vol. 19, no. 3, Sept. 1990, pp. 31–44.

Woel85a Woelk, D., and Luther, W., "Multimedia Database Requirements – Rev.0," MCC Technical Report no. DB-042-85, Austin, Texas, 1985.

Woel86a Woelk, D., Kim, W., and Luther, W., "An Object-Oriented Approach to Multimedia Databases," in *Proc. ACM SIGMOD '86 Int. Conf. on Management of Data* (Washington, D.C., May 1986), ed. C. Zaniolo, also *ACM SIGMOD Record,* vol. 15, no. 2, June 1986, pp. 311–325.

Woel87a Woelk, D., and Kim, W., "Multimedia Information Management in an Object-Oriented Database System," in *Proc. Int. Conf. on VLDB* (Brighton, England, Sept. 1987).

Towards the Modelling of Multimedia Environments: From the Image/Audio Signals to the Documents

Georg Rainer Hofmann and Rüdiger Strack

Fraunhofer Institute for Computer Graphics (IGD)
Wilhelminenstraße 7, D–6100 Darmstadt, Germany

1 Introduction

The ongoing technical development of image communication and interchange, general–purpose computer graphics workstations, as well as personal computers equipped with special–purpose image display hardware, plays a role of increasing importance. This field of image communication has been described in a previous report [12] — with respect to the background of the three scientific disciplines

- telecommunication engineering,
- electrical engineering, and
- computer science.

In these disciplines, various standards for image communication and interchange have been already developed. Unfortunately, the standards most often have been elaborated separately and in isolation from each other. Also, terminology has been developed in the different disciplines such that the same terms are used to mean different things. Therefore, the relevant terminology, encompassing terms like

(1) image model,
(2) image signal,
(3) image format,
(4) image data structure,
(5) digital image/discrete image,
(6) geometric resolution of digital images, or
(7) video/moving picture

has been examined in [12] and related to each other in a basic model. The algorithms respectively devices, either realized in software or hardware, as required, e.g., for

> image acquisition, image storage, image (de)compression, image display, or image (signal or document) transmission and interchange,

developed by the above–mentioned disciplines of science, have been set into relation, guided by a basic image model.
A general, comprehensive framework for imaging and image communication has been elaborated in [28]. This framework, called *Image Communication Open Architecture*, encompasses the various requirements of the entire field of imaging and image communication. Within this framework, various standards for imaging and image communication may be related. For the establishment of this framework, the basic ideas of the model provided by [12] have been discussed and included as a processing perspective.
This report concentrates, by further development of the basic ideas provided by [12], on the relation of the various derivatives of image representations (types) to other media, namely audio. The report also gives some remarks on the synchronization of image data (i.e., in most cases, video data) and audio data. Synchronization in this respect means both spatial and temporal relationship.

2 From the image/audio signal to the documents

There are many reasons that the data type "image" is being considered the most important one within multimedia environments.
Therefore, first the variety of image representations (types) is examined.
The 'evolution' of the image signal to the image document is considered to take place in eight stages, namely

(A) the optical image signal,
(B) the analog image signal,
(C) the digital image signal,
(D) the raw image data bit stream,
(E) the image data structure (raw pixel array), oriented towards real–time display
(E') the image data structure (raw pixel array), oriented towards document structures
(F) the image data interchange format,
(G) the image within document interchange formats, and
(H) the image within interpersonal messages.

These eight types of image representation will be examined with respect to the following questions:

1. What are the characteristic features of the image types (A) to (H)?
2. Which processes transform one image type into another, and vice versa?
3. How can the various image types be processed?
4. What is the underlying (tele-)communication mechanism for the various image types?

ternal structure might be, e.g., a block structure or a (document) page structure. Pixel arrays may well be stored in files, although some image data structures are still defining a fixed data bandwidth with which they have to be transmitted — this is illustrated by dividing the image (E) in subcategories (E) and (E') in Figure 1. Examples are the image data structure for audiovisual services (e.g., video conference) according to CCITT Rec. H.261 [10], or the binary pixel array of the facsimile service according to CCITT Rec. T.4 [3] and T.6 [4]. Other examples are the input image data structures of compression schemata, like MPEG, i.e. MPEG-video [16], JBIG [18], and JPEG [14].

(F) The image data interchange format:
'Image data interchange formats' are designed to serve as file formats for the storage of digital images. In contrast to the image types (A) through (E), image data interchange formats show a generalization of the image parameters. Thus, most image data interchange formats are able to serve as a storage or interchange means for a very large variety of different parameterized images. Image interchange formats are specified by giving their syntax. The encoding of the image data should be separated from the syntax of the data format to provide hardware-independence. A suitable standard which supports the independence between syntax and encoding is the ISO/IEC and CCITT standard ASN.1 [8] which defines an abstract syntax notation. Also, encoding rules for syntax entities specified in ASN.1 are provided in form of the BER [9]. Indeed, the *Image Interchange Facility* (IIF) [19], as Part 3 of ISO/IEC 12087, a comprehensive image data interchange format uses ASN.1. Other examples of image data interchange formats are TIFF [1], and the envelope of JPEG, JFIF.

There are some image types referred to as 'image file formats' that are rather straight memory dumps of the frame buffer of a monitor system, or that exactly reflect the characteristics of a single camera or sensor system. This kind of inflexible image file format would be better referred to as 'pixel arrays', as described above as image type (E).

(G) The image within document interchange formats:
Since the image types (A) through (F) describe — in most cases — iconic data only, there is a need to handle image data in conjunction with other data types, such as text, audio, graphics, etc. Moreover, there is a need to define the layout structure of a document, which is actually the desired results of the rendering process of a document. Therefore, document interchange formats define a framework in which different so-called content types may be incorporated for interchange. A typical example is the *Open Document Architecture* (ODA) [21]. ODA:89 incorporates the *Raster Graphics Content Architecture* (RGCA) which is restricted to a facsimile binary pixel array as image content type.

(H) The image within interpersonal messages:

Document interchange formats — as described above as image type (G) — are, in turn, incorporated into 'interpersonal messages'. These interpersonal messages are treated by message handling services. Roughly speaking, these services emulate the postal service of sending and delivering letters, by electronic means. An example is the ***Message Handling System*** (MHS) according to CCITT Rec. X.400 [5].

Image type (H) may also encompass other existing communication standards which can be used for the transfer of documents. E.g. documents might be incorporated into DTAM [11] or FTAM [20].

2.2 Which processes transform one image type into another and vice versa?

From the optical image signal (A) to the analog image signal (B):

This process is performed by electro–optical (opto–electronic, respectively) conversion. Devices to perform these conversions are monitor systems, typically equipped with cathode ray tubes, camera systems, and the like. Basic parameters of an image, as fields per second or lines per field, appear as device–specific constants.

From the analog image signal (B) to the digital image signal (C):

This process is called analog/digital conversion (A/D and D/A conversion, respectively). In case of image signal analog/digital conversion, sampling and quantization have to take place. The continuous presentation of an (analog) image line is transformed into a discrete presentation. In the digital image, the line consists of discrete pixels.

From the digital image signal (C) to the raw image data bit stream (D):

This process is a basic encoding of the amplitude values of the pixels, lines, etc., of the digital image signal. The encoding process selects, among others, the numbers of bits per pixel value, as well as the semantics of these values against colormetric measures.

From the raw image data bit stream (D) to the image data structure (raw pixel array) (E):

This process adds some more structuring capabilities, e.g., blocks, array structures, group–of–blocks, etc., to the image data bit stream. Moreover, this process selects a finite interval from the — potentially endless — raw image data bit stream.

From the image data structure (raw pixel array) (E) to the image data interchange format (F):

This process performs a 'generalization' of the major/typical image parameters. The inverse process is the instantiation of the image data interchange format by (application–) specific parameters of an image. From the image data interchange format (F) to the image within document interchange formats (G): This process performs an integration of the (iconic) image interchange formats into overall document architectures.

The inverse process — an integral part of the so-called 'document formatter' programs — performs an 'unwrapping' of the image data, and finally leads to the display of the unwrapped image.

From the image within document interchange formats (G) to the image within interpersonal messages (H):
This process performs an integration of the image interchange formats or the document interchange formats into an interpersonal message structure, as used in message handling systems.

2.3 How can the various image types be processed?

(A) The optical image signal:
Almost no possibilities of 'processing' optical image signals by digital computers are given.

(B) The analog image signal:
Processing takes place by analog (or hybrid) processors, often referred to as 'filters.' These devices may, e.g., alter the image's basic parameters by geometric (spatial) or temporal resampling.

(C) The digital image signal:
Basically the same as what is said under (B) applies: Processing takes place by digital processors, often referred to as 'digital filters.' These devices may, e.g., alter the image's basic parameters by geometrical (spatial) or temporal resampling. This process is sometimes also referred to as 'image format transcoding.'

(D) The raw image data bit stream, and (E) the image data structure (raw pixel array):
At these levels, compression algorithms and processes typically take place. Here, lossless arithmetic coding algorithms and lossy transform codings deal with image data bit streams and pixel arrays. In this field, a number of internationally standardized compression schemata and algorithms have been developed. Among these are the well-known algorithms JPEG, JBIG, MPEG-video [16], etc. For an overview about compression schemata see e.g. [29] or [27].

(F) The image data interchange format:
Like other syntax-wise defined information entities (like programming languages), image interchange formats are generated, parsed, and interpreted by comprehensive software tools. Different image data interchange formats are converted into each other, under software control. This latter process is sometimes referred to as 'image conversion.'

(G) The image within document interchange formats:
Image contents in document architectures undergo processes of editing, layout, and rendering.

(H) The image within interpersonal messages:
Interpersonal messages are treated in open communication environments. These processes are not image-specific at all.

2.4 What is the underlying (tele–)communication mechanism for the various image types?

(A) The optical image signal:
This image type — actually a two–dimensional visible image — can hardly be transmitted electronically.

(B) The analog image signal:
This image type is typically emitted in broadcast systems and environments, such as TV signal broadcasting by satellites, or in cables.

(C) The digital image signal; and (D) the raw image data bit stream:
These image types might be broadcasted by digital TV broadcasting, comparable to image type (B).

(E) The image data structure (raw pixel array):
These image formats are used by a variety of telecommunication services; some of them are internationally standardized. The main feature of these services is that they are defined relatively close to the carrying network. This holds for the audiovisual conferencing services, e.g. H.261, as well as for the facsimile document transmission services, i.e. CCITT Rec. T.4 and T.6.

(F) The image data interchange format, the (G) image within document interchange formats, and (H) the image within interpersonal messages:
These items are communicated in open environments, whereas most of them are designed by applying the OSI reference model according to CCITT Rec. X.200 [6]. Typically, they cover layer 7 of OSI and are syntactically defined by means belonging to layer 6 of OSI.

2.5 Relationship of image types (A) to (H) to audio formats

According to Figure 1, there is an audio–oriented reference model which may be compared against the eight–stage model of the image types. This audio model is shown in Figure 2. In this figure, the following analogies are shown:

(A) The audio signal 'sound' corresponds to the optical image signal.

(B) The analog audio signal corresponds to the analog image signal.

(C) The digital audio signal corresponds to the digital image signal.

(D) The audio data bit stream, e.g., according to CCITT Rec. G.711 [7], corresponds to the raw image data bit stream.

(E) Some audio data structures and documents, like CD [13], MPEG–audio [17], etc., correspond to the image data structure (raw pixel array), and the subsequent stages (F) to (H) of the eight–stage model of Figure 1.

The characteristic features of these audio type can be outlined — according to the definitions of Section 2.1 — as follows:

(A) The audio signal 'sound':
The acoustical 'sound' audio signal (A) is the only audio type which

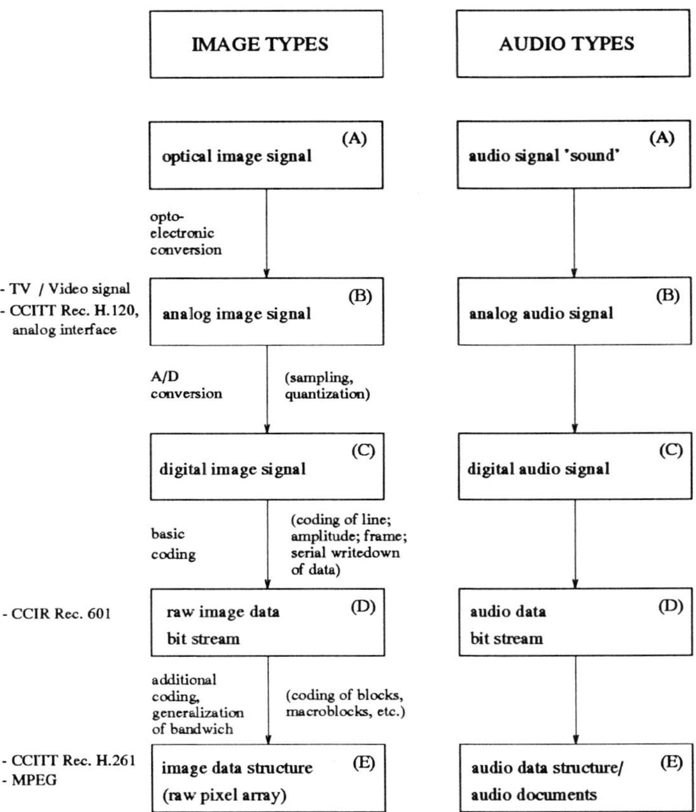

Fig. 2. Different audio types (A) to (E)

can be heard directly by the human ear. This signal may be understood physically as small alterations of air pressure in the environment. However, comparable to the interpretation of visual information by the human eye, the interpretation of sonic information by the human ear system is a highly complicated process.

(B) The analog audio signal:
The so–called 'analog audio signal' can be characterized as a function of voltage over time. Almost all known audio signals — in contrast to the image signals — are one–dimensional signals. A typical example is an audio signal, as taken in by microphones.

(C) The digital audio signal:
The digital audio signal is based on a certain sampling frequency, and certain quantization steps. The quantization steps determine the resolution with which the amplitude values of the audio signal are quantized.

(D) The audio data bit stream:
The audio data bit stream is a raw sequence of encoded amplitude values of a digital audio signal. An important and typical parameter of an audio data bit stream is its data rate. This is the amount of data that has to be transferred per second. A typical example of an audio data bit stream is the digital audio format according to CCITT Rec. G.711. This standard, however, also encompasses prescriptions for the sampling and quantization of analog audio signals to digital audio signals.

(E) Audio data structures and documents:
These audio types, e.g. CD, MPEG–audio, most often, appear as finite sets of audio data. Thus, this audio type is in contrast to the other audio types which appear as potentially infinite audio signals. This fact may well be analogous to the distinction of image types (A) to (E), and (E') to (H), respectively. See Section 2.1 for further explanations.

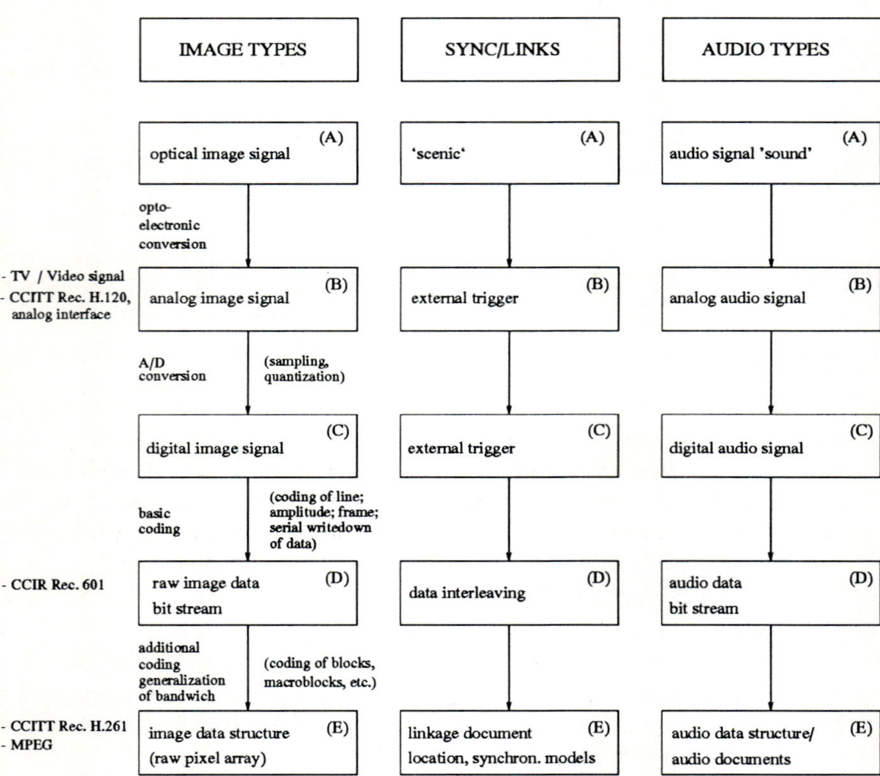

Fig. 3. Synchronization mechanisms for image and audio

2.6 Relationship and synchronization of image types (A) to (H) with other media

In addition to the reference model, as shown in Figure 2, the mechanisms of synchronization and linking of image and audio data may be outlined as shown in 3. The synchronization mechanisms may be outlined as follows:

(A) The linking of audio signal 'sound' to the optical image signal:
There is hardly any technology–oriented mechanism for synchronization and/or linking at all. Instead, if these two 'information types' shall be synchronized, this only can be achieved 'manually', based on their scenic contents.

(B) The linking of analog audio signal to the analog image signal:
This kind is typically achieved by means of an external trigger mechanism. Such an external mechanism — which may be seen as a separate standard — is, e.g., the SMPTE time code mechanism.

(C) The linking of the digital audio signal to the digital image signal:
Here holds essentially the same as outlined under item (B) above.

(D) The linking of audio data bit stream, e.g., according to CCITT Rec. G.711, to the raw image data bit stream:
Here, the linking between the two data types is achieved in most cases by 'data interleaving'. This means, that the image data and the audio data — when forming an audio–image data stream — are combined. For example, within a certain time interval of the audio–image signal, all audiovisual data is contained in the data stream.

(E) The linking of audio data structures and audio documents to the image data structure (raw pixel array), and the subsequent stages (F) to (H):
As a general guideline different media such as character text, geometric graphics, images and audio, should overlap in functionality as little as possible. Multimedia and hypermedia structuring capabilities should be the *glue* which combine these common types both in space and time. Various international standardization efforts concentrate on these aspects providing general mechanisms to relate media to each other. These mechanisms appear to have highly sophisticated semantics. For example, the standards HyTime [24], HyperODA [22] [23] and MHEG [25] do include such sophisticated mechanisms by providing location and synchronization models.
Nevertheless, if the respective multimedia/hypermedia architecture does not permit to map synchronization information existing between separate audio and image structures in the interchange format a separate image–audio representation type is necessary. MPEG can be used as an example for the latter. The MPEG–system [15] provides for the interlinking respective combination of image data structures (MPEG–video) and audio data structures (MPEG–audio) in order to form a single data stream, which is more adapted to digital image storage or transmission.

3 Levels of integration of different media into multimedia workstations

3.1 Rendering and display of multimedia data types (A) to (H)

The rendering of multimedia data is commonly closely associated with the 'display' process of images. The basic model may be seen as

> Image Type (A) to (H) ⟶ Image Rendering and Display ⟶ (Human) Observer

which, in turn, is the basic model of any rendering and display pipeline. For the following reasons, the image rendering and display process turns out to be rather complex:

1. Due to the physical nature, only image types (A) — according to Figure 1 — can be seen by a human observer.
2. An image rendering or display process may accept image types other than (A). But, due to the previous fact, the different stages of image types must be passed until stage (A) has been reached. For example, if the rendering process accepts an image interchange format (type (F) in Figure 1), then
   - the pixel arrays (type (E) in Figure 1) must be isolated;
   - they must be transformed into a bit stream (type (D) in Figure 1), which, in turn, may be stored in the frame buffer of the system;
   - whereas this bit stream is read out of the frame buffer as a digital image signal (type (C) in Figure 1) by a video controller.
   - The video controller produces an analog image signal (type (B) in Figure 1), and
   - finally, the analog signal is transformed into a visible optical image signal (type (A) in Figure 1) by a monitor system or any other display device.
3. The different stages of the rendering process, as outlined under the previous item, may be highly incompatible. Thus, extensive resampling of the iconic image data must be made. Besides, hardware restrictions may play a major role. For example, the rendering of an image array of a larger size than the size of the monitor's frame buffer requires an alteration of the image size prior to display.
4. The dimension of time — as the most important component of the moving pictures — is a separate issue. Due to drawbacks of parts of the current technology, the required data rates, as well as the sensity of the human observer to display errors and the rendering of moving pictures — especially on the platform of computer graphics workstations – has now different technical solutions. These are described in the following section.

3.2 Different display/rendering architectures

In Section 2 and Figure 1, different stages of the evolution from the image signal to the image document have been identified. In Section 3.1 as outlined under item (2), it has been shown that the image rendering process has to successively transform the different stages of the image types (H) through (A), until a visible (optical) presentation of the image is achieved. In telecommunication terminals and in computer graphics workstations or personal computers, the image rendering process is mapped onto specific architectural features of the computer system. These specific architectural features form display pipelines consisting of different stages. The integration of image rendering is quite different; it depends on the layer of integration of the image data with the other data that is handled by the computer system. The typical layers of integration may be classified as follows; see also Figure 4 for illustration:

(i) Optical layer,
(ii) electronic layer,
(iii) frame buffer layer,
(iv) data structure layer, and
(v) document layer.

In the following paragraphs, these layers of integration are briefly described and characterized.

(i) Optical layer:
This (trivial case) integration of image display on this layer is optically performed. Different monitor and/or projection systems are arranged in such a way that the (human) observer is able to look at these different displays simultaneously. Some different images and other data may be optically combined. No common processing of image data and other computer data takes place.

(ii) Electronic layer:
At this layer of integration, the analog signal of the image is combined with the video input signals of the workstations' monitor system. This may be performed using, e.g., the chroma–key technique. The user at the workstation user interface may manipulate the displayed image — that appears in a window at the user interface — only to a very limited extent. The placement of the image on the screen may be altered. However, the image data is only displayed; it usually can not be read into the computer's main memory. This kind of integration is also referred to as 'video in windows'. It is important to note that this layer does not exist for some systems. These are systems with special display devices whose input is not an analog electronic signal, e.g., plasma panels or LCD screens.

(iii) Frame buffer layer:
In this case of integration, the workstation's frame buffer is directly accessed by the display hardware. The user at the workstation interface

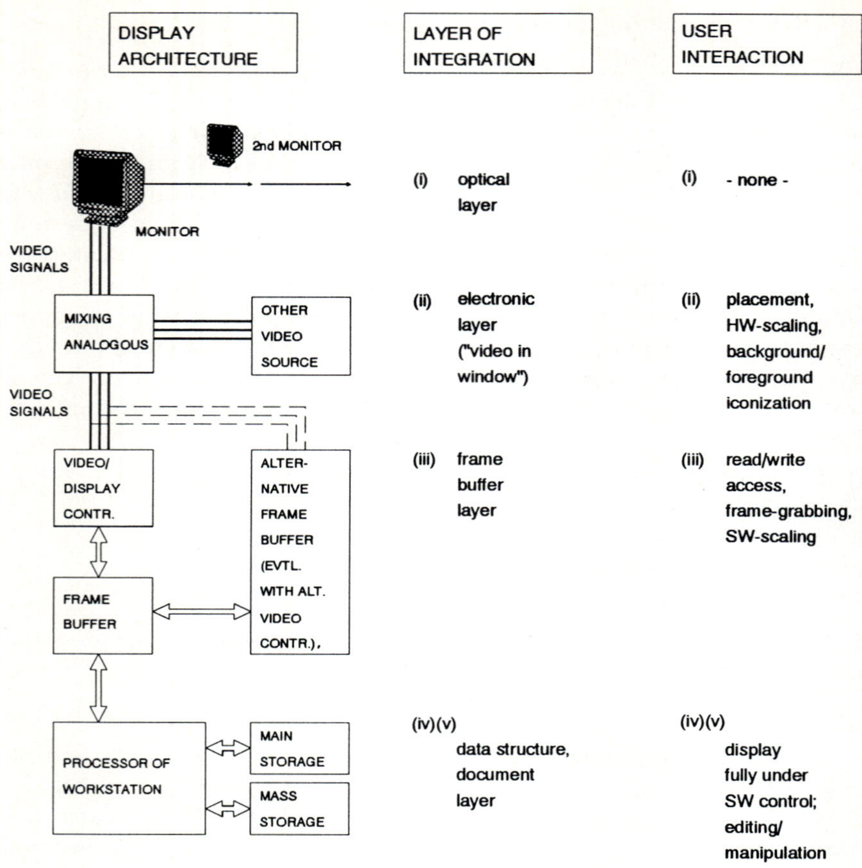

Fig. 4. Levels of integration of images in multimedia workstation display systems

may perform some interaction with the displayed image data structure. The image may be placed, scaled, etc. Some pixel arrays of the displayed image, including single fields of a displayed moving picture, can be read out of the frame buffer into the workstation's internal memory. It is important to note that this layer does not exist for some systems. These are systems with no directly accessible frame buffer at all. However, special-purpose display hardware, as added to personal computers, may emulate the functionality of a frame buffer.

(iv) Data structure layer:

At this layer of integration, images are handled as instantiations of image data structures. Images are stored, processed, and displayed under full (software) control of the processor of the computer system. Moving pictures are displayed via frame-per-frame rendering through the full display pipeline that is formed by the computer's mass storage, the main processor, the frame buffer, and the regular computer monitor system. In case of moving pictures, additional features like fully parameterized display field frequency at the user interface are realized, under software control.

(v) Document layer:
The integration at this layer allows for the full manipulation of the image data. The document data, including the image data, may be edited and revised by appropriate software systems, also referred to as 'document editors.'

In general, it is possible to state that the historical technical development of the integration of image rendering into the regular computer (i.e., computer graphics workstations, as well as PCs) display systems has taken place in the sequence (i) to (v). The integration layer (i) may be considered to be technically trivial, anyway. In the beginning of the 1980s, a technical solution according to integration layer (ii), known as 'video in windows', has been considered as a multimedia system. At the level of integration layer (iii), medium–price PC–based solutions and systems are at hand. Technical systems according to integration layers (iv) and (v) are currently being developed on a prototype basis.

4 Conclusion

By illuminating the situation of image communication and interchange in the context of multimedia systems, the following results have been elaborated:
There is a considerable amount of confusion and ambiguity in the usage of image communication terms and vocabulary. Since a variety of image representation are not differentiated enough — even though they are referring to things that are quite different in nature — a processing perspective respectively a basic model has been elaborated, as shown in Figure 1. With this model, it is possible to duplicate the stages from the image signal to the image document.
This report also provides the relation of the various derivatives of image representations to other media, namely audio. Similar stages have been identified in regard to audio. Especially, the synchronization mechanisms for image and audio have been clarified.
Image display architectures for computers and telecommunication terminals are also dealing with image representations (types). However, these types are quite different in nature. Here, the different technical solutions — being reflected at the various layers of integration of image display, as shown in Section 3.2 — must not be mixed up.
The paper attempts to provide a basic model for the area of image communication and interchange considering the relation to other media, especially audio. This model may be useful in the evaluation process of service components and service primitives for image and multimedia communication, as well

as for the transcoding and migration from different image representations and image communication services.

5 Acknowledgements

The authors would like to thank Susanne Wurster for proof reading, and Norbert Gerfelder for helpful technical comments. The design of the eight–stage model (Figure 1) has been inspired at a certain degree by Detlef Krömker's reference model of visualization systems [26]. Colleagues (Christof Blum, Ralf Cordes, Bob Day, David Duce, Narciso Garcia, Eckhardt Moeller, Dale Sutcliffe and others) from the RACE AMICS project have contributed to this paper in technical discussions.
The work reflected in this paper has been performed within the project *Advanced Multimedia Image Communication Services* (AMICS) (RACE project R2056), supported within the RACE II program by the Commission of the European Communities (CEC).

References

1. Aldus Corporation, Seattle. *Tag Image File Format Specification, Revision 6.0*, 1992.
2. CCIR. *Encoding Parameters of Digital Television for Studios, Recommendation 601/2*, volume XI — Part 1 of *Recommendations of the CCIR*. CCIR, 1990.
3. CCITT. *Standardization of Group 3 Facsimile Apparatus for Document Processing, Recommendation T.4*. Red Book. CCITT, 1984.
4. CCITT. *Facsimile Coding Schemes and Coding Control Functions for Group 4 Facsimile Apparatus, Recommendation T.6*. Blue Book. CCITT, 1988.
5. CCITT. *Message Handling Systems and Service Overview, Recommendation X.400*. Blue Book. CCITT, 1988.
6. CCITT. *Open System Interconnection (OSI), Recommendation X.200*. Blue Book. CCITT, 1988.
7. CCITT. *Pulse Code Modulation of PCM Channels of Voice Frequencies, Recommendation G.711*. Blue Book. CCITT, 1988.
8. CCITT. *Specification of Abstract Syntax Notation One (ASN.1), Recommendation X.208*. Blue Book. CCITT, 1988.
9. CCITT. *Specification of Basic Encoding Rules for Abstract Syntax Notation One (ASN.1), Recommendation X.209*. Blue Book. CCITT, March 1988.
10. CCITT. *Video Codec for Audiovisual Services at p*64 kbit/s, Recommendation H.261*. CCITT, 1990.
11. CCITT. *Document Transfer and Manipulation (DTAM) — Services and Protocols — Introduction and General Principles, Draft Recommendation T.431*. CCITT, September 1992.
12. G.R. Hofmann. The modelling of images for communication in multimedia environments and the evolution from the image signal to the image document. *The Visual Computer*, (9):303–317, 1993.

13. *IEC 908:198 CD Digital Audio System.* IEC.

14. *ISO/IEC DIS 10918: Digital Compression and Coding of Continuous-tone Still Images.* ISO/IEC, 1992.

15. *ISO/IEC DIS 11172-1: Coded Representation of Picture and Audio Information, Coding of Moving Pictures and Associated Audio for Digital Storage Media up to about 1.5 Mbit/s — Part 1: Systems.* ISO/IEC, April 1992.

16. *ISO/IEC DIS 11172-2: Coded Representation of Picture and Audio Information, Coding of Moving Pictures and Associated Audio for Digital Storage Media up to about 1.5 Mbit/s — Part 2: Video.* ISO/IEC, April 1992.

17. *ISO/IEC DIS 11172-3: Coded Representation of Picture and Audio Information, Coding of Moving Pictures and Associated Audio for Digital Storage Media up to about 1.5 Mbit/s — Part 3: Audio.* ISO/IEC, April 1992.

18. *ISO/IEC DIS 11554: Coded Representation of Picture and Audio Information, Progressive Bi-level Image Compression Standard.* ISO/IEC, June 1992.

19. *ISO/IEC DIS 12087-3: Information Technology — Computer Graphics and Image Processing — Image Processing and Interchange (IPI) — Functional Specification — Part 3: Image Interchange Facility (IIF).* ISO/IEC, November 1992.

20. *ISO/IEC IS 8571: Information Processing Systems — Open Systems Interconnection (OSI) — File Transfer, Access and Management (FTAM).* ISO/IEC, 1988.

21. *ISO/IEC IS 8613: Information Processing — Text and Office Systems — Office Document Architecture (ODA) and Interchange Format (ODIF).* ISO/IEC, 1989.

22. *ISO/IEC IS 8613/PDAM 7: Information Processing — Text and Office Systems — Office Document Architecture (ODA) and Interchange Format (ODIF) — Amendment 7: HyperODA — Extensions for Temporal Relationships.* ISO/IEC, 1992.

23. *ISO/IEC IS 8613/PDAM 8: Information Processing — Text and Office Systems — Office Document Architecture (ODA) and Interchange Format (ODIF) — Amendment 8: HyperODA — Extensions for Non-linear Structures.* ISO/IEC, 1992.

24. *ISO/IEC IS 10744: Information Technology — Hypermedia/Time-based Structuring Language (HyTime).* ISO/IEC, 1992.

25. ISO/IEC JTC1/SC29. *Coded Representation of Multimedia and Hypermedia Information Objects, Part 1: Representation and Base Notation WG12 Working Draft WD 0.0.* ISO/IEC, December 1992.

26. D. Krömker. Visualisierungssysteme. PhD Thesis, TH Darmstadt, Darmstadt, 1991.

27. J. Maurer editor. Digital Multimedia Systems. *Communications of the ACM*, 34(4), April 1991.

28. R. Strack editor, C. Blum, R. Cordes, I. Defée, D.A. Duce, N. García, G.R. Hofmann, R. Maybury, E. Moeller, M.J. Pérez-Luque, D.C. Sutcliffe, and R. Strack. Conceptual Building Blocks for an Image Communication Open Architecture (ICOA). Deliverable R2056/FhG/IGD/DS/P/002/b1, RACE Project R2056 Advanced Multimedia Image Communication Services (AMICS), April 1993.

29. H. Yasuda. Standardization activities on multimedia coding in ISO. *Signal Processing: Image Communication*, 1(1):3–16, 1989.

A Glossary

ASN.1:	Abstract Syntax Notation One
BER:	Basic Encoding Rules
CAI:	Common Architecture for Imaging
CIF:	Common Intermediate Format
DTAM:	Document Transfer and Manipulation
FTAM:	File Transfer, Access and Management
HDTV:	High Definition Television
HyTime:	Hypermedia/Time–based Document Representation Language
HyperODA	Hyper ODA
IIF:	Image Interchange Facility
IPI:	Image Processing and Interchange
JBIG:	Joint Bilevel Image Group
JFIF:	JPEG File Interchange Format
JPEG:	Joint Photographic Experts Group
MHS:	Message Handling System
MHEG:	Multimedia and Hypermedia Information coding Experts Group
MPEG:	Motion Picture coding Experts Group
ODA:	Office/Open Document Architecture
ODIF:	Office Document Interchange Format
OSI:	Open System Interconnection
PCM:	Pulse Code Modulation
RACE:	Research and Development in Advanced Communications Technologies in Europe
RGCA:	Raster Graphics Content Architecture
Rec.:	Recommendation
RLE:	Run–Length Encoding
SMPTE:	Society of Motion Picture and Television Engineers
TIFF:	Tagged Image File Format
TV:	Television

This article was processed using the LaTeX macro package with LMAMULT style

Integration of Motion Video into Multimedia Computers

B. Girod
Lehrstuhl für Nachrichtentechnik, Universität Erlangen-Nürnberg
Cauerstraße 7, D-91058 Erlangen, Germany

1 Introduction

Computers were originally invented as programable calculation engines. Today, they are evolving more and more into universal, flexible communication platforms. Multimedia computers that integrate text, graphics, audio and images will be one the important developments of this decade. Motion video is a particularly powerful modality of multimedia communications; unfortunately, it also poses the greatest technical difficulties. Before motion video can be integrated into computers, several related problems have yet to be solved. These include issues in the areas of video signal representation and system architecture, and they are coupled by the real-time constraint of motion video. In this contribution, I discuss some of the key problems and possible solutions for the integration of motion video and computers.

Section 2 reviews some typical applications of the combination of motion video and computers which will be referred to later. Section 3 discusses the benefits of digitally integrated motion video vs. analog video disks. Section 4 is devoted to video data compression with special attention paid to the MPEG standard. Scalable video is discussed in section 5, while delay issues are the subject of section 6.

2 Applications of Computer-Integrated Motion Video

Among the first interactive video disks was the "Aspen Movie Map", produced at MIT's Architecture Machine Group in 1978. The group had driven through the town of Aspen, Colorado, and recorded views in four directions approximately every 3 meters. The pictures were stored on an analog video disk and could be played interactively to provide a "surrogate travel" experience. The surrogate traveller would virtually drive through town and could choose to turn at every intersection. Selected buildings could be entered. A button allowed switching between summer and winter views [1] [2].

As their next interactive video disk project, the "Movie Manual," the same group produced an interactive car and bicycle repair manual [1] [2]. At the time, this was another pioneering application. The repair manual was a true hypermedia system, integrating text, annotated graphics, and motion video. User interaction happened via a touch-sensitive screen. Motion video was used to demonstrate certain manual skills and procedures for assembly and disassembly of parts. For example, one movie showed the disastrous result of unscrewing the bolts of the oil pan too quickly: its contents would spill over the mechanic [1].

As a third application scenario, consider computer-supported cooperative work (CSCW) [3]. As shown in Fig. 1, videoconference windows can be incorporated into the window system on the computer screen to allow for on-line audiovisual communication between workstation users. The participants of such a computer videoconference would possibly discuss a spreadsheet which they all share in another window, or they would use a "shared whiteboard" window for sketching and handwriting.

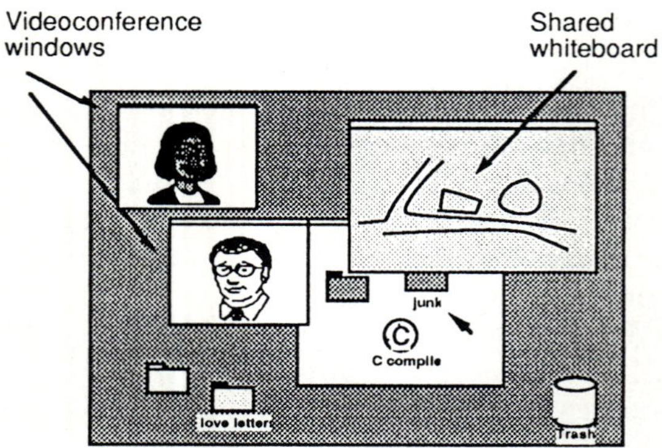

Fig. 1. CSCW with multipoint videoconference and shared whiteboard area.

The market for multimedia systems and services is expected to grow rapidly. Recent studies indicate that the annual market volume will grow by a factor of 5 over the next three years, reaching almost 2500 million ECU in Western Europe and almost 6000 million ECU in the United States by the year 1995 [4]. It is expected that 10-15% of this market will be in the area of office communication, where the CSCW example above might be typical. Another 25-30% will be in marketing and sales applications. In this area, surrogate travel offered by your local travel agent as might serve as an example. The interactive repair manual is representative of education and training, which is expected to constitute another 25-30% of the multimedia market. Finally, the consumer market is expected to constitute another 25-30%.

3 Digital Video in Multimedia Computers

Early interactive video applications used analog video disk players that could be controlled by a computer. Figure 2 shows a block diagram of such a system. A graphics workstation or a personal computer contains a central processing unit (CPU) with random access memory (RAM). Raster graphics is generated by a dedicated raster display processor which is also responsible for refreshing the screen from a frame buffer. The workstation reacts to inputs from devices such as a keyboard or a mouse. A hard disk serves as a mass storage system. The workstation is connected to a local area network (LAN), such as Ethernet, to communicate with other workstations, file servers or peripheral devices. The workstation controls a video disk player such that access to every stored picture is possible with only short delay. The video signal at the output of the disk player is inserted into a rectangular window of the raster display. This is accomplished by chroma keying or by inserting the digitized video signal into the frame buffer. Many multimedia systems with motion video today still use this principle.

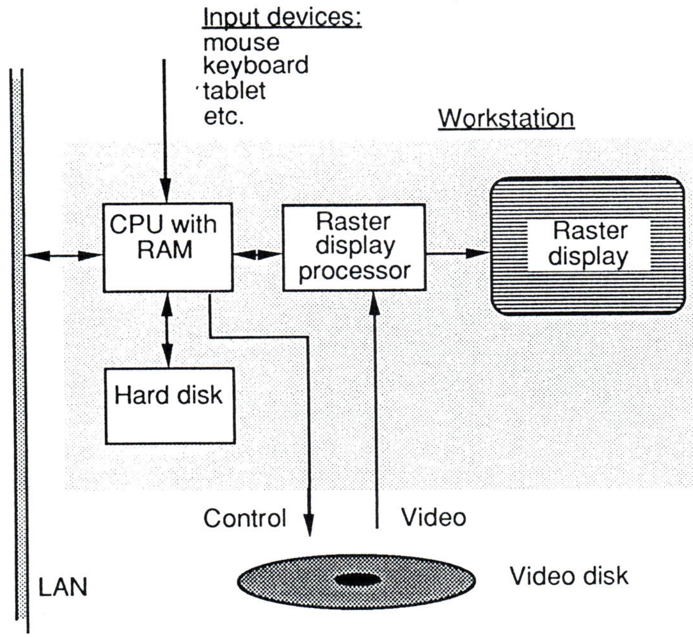

Fig. 2. Workstation with analog video disk

The analog video disk solution described above is not satisfactory in many respects. An analog video disk player is bulky and adds extra expense to the system. Each interactive video workstation needs a dedicated video disk player; there is no way of playing video from a remote server. Unless we digitize the analog video signal, it is not possible to copy video over the LAN or manipulate the video data with our computer.

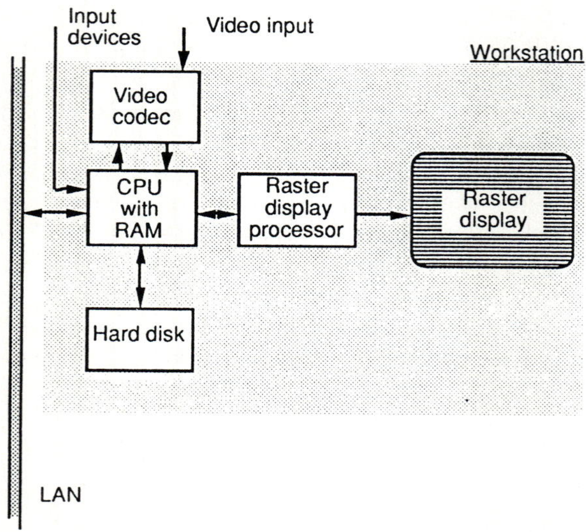

Fig. 3. Workstation with integrated digital video

All these drawbacks can be overcome by integrating digital motion video into the workstation (Fig. 3). Rather than adding an analog video disk player, the system contains a dedicated coprocessor powerful enough to compress and decompress video in real-time. This video codec can be used in various modes:

- For interactive video applications (such as the Movie Manual described in section 2), we store compressed digital video on the hard disk. To play motion video, these data are decompressed and written into the frame store.
- For videoconferencing (such as described in the CSCW scenario in section 2), a camera signal is digitized and fed into the video coder directly. The compressed data are then transmitted over the LAN. Simultaneously, one or several compressed video data streams are received over the LAN, decompressed by the video codec coprocessor and displayed in one or several windows.
- In a video server application, a local workstation would access compressed video stored on the hard disk of a remote server over the LAN. These data would be decompressed and displayed locally.

The major problem with fully integrating motion video into workstations or personal computers is data compression. For example, the digital television studio standard set by CCIR in their recommendation 601 requires sampling rates of 13.5 MHz for the luminance signal Y, and 6.75 MHz for the color difference signals R-Y and B-Y [5]. With an amplitude quantization to 256 levels (or 8 bit), an overall data rate of 216 Mbit/s results. The data rate for an uncompressed HDTV signal is in the order of 1 Gbit/s. Most of today's workstation screens already have a spatial resolution closer to HDTV rather than to standard television. Compare these rates to those handled in current computer systems. A magnetic hard disk will typically allow read and write access at rates up to 10 Mbit/s. An optical compact disk can be read at 1.5 Mbit/s. Ethernet typically allows peak transfer rates up to 10 Mbit/s, but of course the sustained rate depends on the network traffic and is much lower. Local area networks for personal computers might have an even lower peak rate, such as the Apple LocalTalk network with a peak rate of 256 kbit/s. ISDN is becoming widely available now, but its basic channel rate is only 64 kbit/s. Digital video signals have to be compressed substantially to be stored and transmitted at these rates.

In addition to highly efficient data compression, several other requirements have to be met, some of which are general, others are specific to computer integration. Particularly, these include:

- *Picture quality.* Good spatial resolution, sufficient motion rendition, and the absence of compression artifacts are required. For many applications, a picture quality like the one provided by a VHS tape is sufficient, but a better picture quality would of course be preferred.
- *Low delay.* Videoconferencing applications require a low delay, otherwise the interaction between participants is seriously disturbed. For interactive video applications, such as the Aspen Movie Map, short latency is desirable as well.
- *Scalability.* Scalability allows for resizing of a picture in a window system and for graceful degradation in the case of LAN overload or fluctuations in available compute power.
- *Access features.* Fast forward and reverse (with visible picture), slow motion, and freeze frame features should be supported. Random access to individual frames is highly desirable.
- *Editability.* Ideally, we would like to cut and assemble video with the computer on the compressed bit-stream level, but decoding and re-coding of data right before and after a scene cut might be acceptable as well.

4 Video Compression

Video compression is a mature field with an enormous body of literature today. We can only discuss some aspects that are important in the context of integration of motion video into multimedia computers here. Readers with a deeper interest are referred to one of the comprehensive books [6] [7].

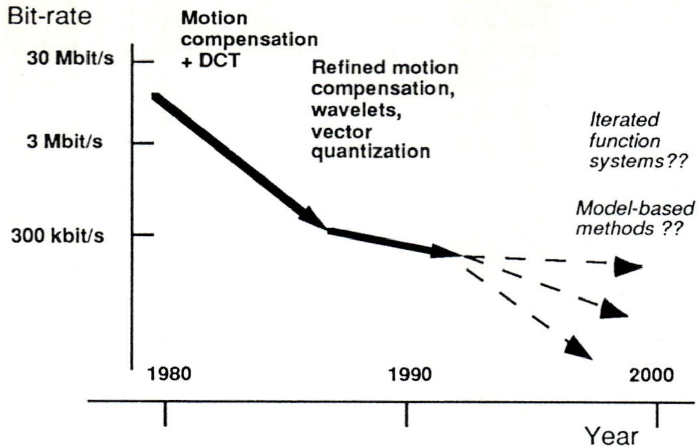

Fig. 4. Bit-rate required to encode motion video with VHS quality

Figure 4 illustrates the progress in motion video compression since 1980. Around 1980, codecs combining motion compensation and the Discrete Cosine Transform (DCT) first appeared [8]. This basic "hybrid coding system" was analyzed, refined and optimized by many different contributors. Lateron, it was found that other signal decompositions, such as the Discrete Wavelet Transform, are superior to the DCT, and vector quantization can outperform scalar quantization, as is typically used with the DCT [9] [10]. Still, today's video compression standards are based on a combination of motion compensation and DCT coding. The rate required to encode a full motion video signal at VHS quality has come down from around 20 Mbit/s to well below 1 Mbit/s today (end 1992). For head-and-shoulder views typical for videoconferencing, rates can be substantially lower still. As algorithms are maturing, it has become harder and harder to lower the data rate even further. For the existing schemes, there is probably little room for improvement. New approaches, such as compression with iterated functions systems [11] or "model-based coding" [12] have yet to prove that they can lead to results superior to the classical waveform coding algorithms. It is doubtful whether bit-rate reduction for the VHS quality level can be advanced by another order of magnitude in the future.

Motion compensation and DCT coding are the basis for the MPEG-1 video compression standard. MPEG is the "Moving Picture Experts Group" of the International Standards Organization (ISO). The MPEG-1 development was finished in 1991 [13] [14]. While it is not limited to the storage of motion video on compact disk, this application played an important role in the development of the standard. Bit-rate and image size can be set flexibly, but typical parameters are 1.5 Mbit/s (including multiple compressed audio channels) and an image size of 288 lines x 352 pels. Frame rate is between 24 and 30 Hz. Unlike current television standards, MPEG-1 does not include line-interlace, so that display on non-interlaced computer screens is easily possible. Currently, the group is developing the MPEG-2 standard, targeted at interlaced material and higher bit-rates. MPEG-2 is supposed to be set in 1994. The picture quality target is NTSC, PAL, or SECAM quality at 3 - 5 Mbit/s, and at least MAC (multiplexed analog components) quality at 10 Mbit/s. MPEG-2 will probably have some compatibility with MPEG-1, as well as with the CCITT Recommendation H.26x currently under development for the transmission of video over ATM (asynchronous transfer mode) networks.

The similarity of successive frames in a video sequence is exploited by the MPEG algorithm, utilizing motion-compensated prediction [15]. Rather than encoding each frame by itself, changes from frame to frame are encoded. If the luminance of the frame to be encoded can be predicted precisely from previously transmitted frames, the required bit-rate is low. In order to reduce the prediction error as much as possible, the frame-to-frame displacement is measured and used for prediction. The displacement vector field is also needed for decoding and therefore transmitted as "side information." The principle of motion-compensated prediction is illustrated in Figure 5.

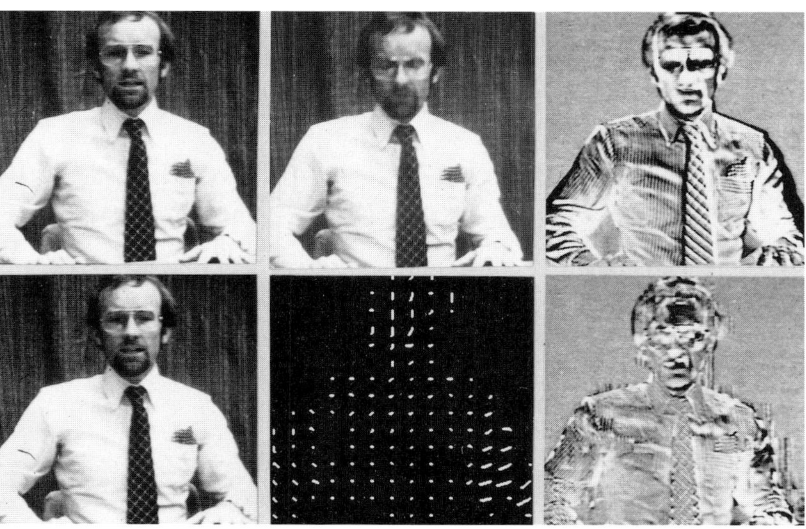

Fig. 5. Principle of motion-compensated prediction. Successive frames can be encoded independently (top row, first two pictures), or the pel-wise frame-to-frame difference is encoded (top row, third picture). To reduce the frame difference further, motion compensation is used, but the displacement vector field has to be transmitted as "side information" (bottom row).

Motion-compensated prediction can be incorporated into different data structures to represent sequences of images. The simplest strategy is used, for example, in CCITT Recommendation H.261 for encoding of videotelephony signals at multiples of 64 kbit/s [16] [20]. This standard preceeded MPEG. With the H.261 scheme, the first frame is encoded in intraframe mode, i.e., without reference to other frames in the sequence. Then, as illustrated in Figure 6, all successive frames are encoded in their natural order, using the preceeding frame for prediction. In principle, this strategy can lead to a codec with minimum delay. Unfortunately, it supports none of the access features required in section 3. If a video sequence has been encoded and stored according to H.261, all previous frames have to be read and decoded to access an individual frame. Random access is not possible, nor is fast forward or reverse operation with a visible picture.

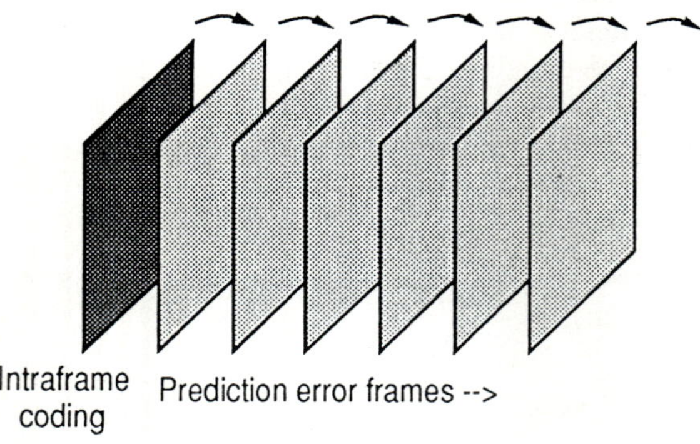

Fig. 6. Frame structure in CCITT H.261.

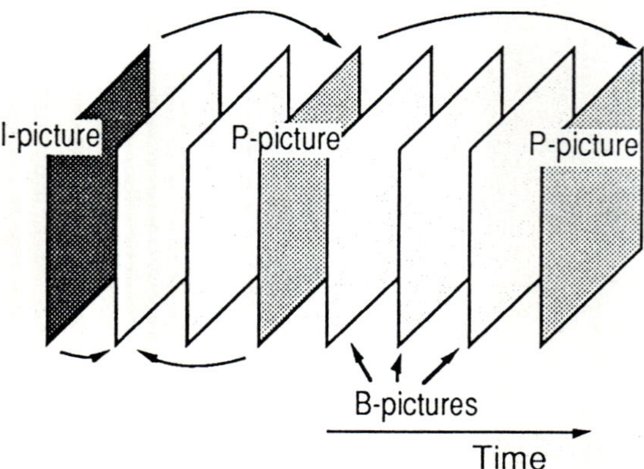

Fig. 7. Hierarchical frame structure in MPEG-1

MPEG-1 overcomes the access difficulties built into H.261 by using the hierarchical frame structure shown in Figure 7. The encoder can declare frames to be one of three types. *I-pictures* are encoded in intraframe mode, i.e., by themselves. *P-pictures* are predicted from the previous I-picture or P-picture. *B-pictures* are predicted from a closest past I-picture or P-picture and the closest future I-picture or P-picture. The "B" in B-picture stands for bidirectional prediction. Each potential entry point in the sequence should be encoded as an I-picture. Typically, there would always be a few B-pictures between P-pictures or I-pictures. For fast forward operation, one would skip some or all of the B-pictures. Fast reverse operation can either only use the I-pictures, or move backwards through sequences of I- and P-pictures, but play each of these sequences in fast forward mode. When encoding with MPEG-1, one has to find the right trade-off between random access capability and efficient data compression. With many I-pictures, coding efficiency drops since I-pictures do not exploit their similarity to other pictures. Having many successive B-pictures introduces a large coding delay. For decoding, this is not an issue, since the frames are transmitted or stored in the order that they are needed for decoding, rather than in chronological order.

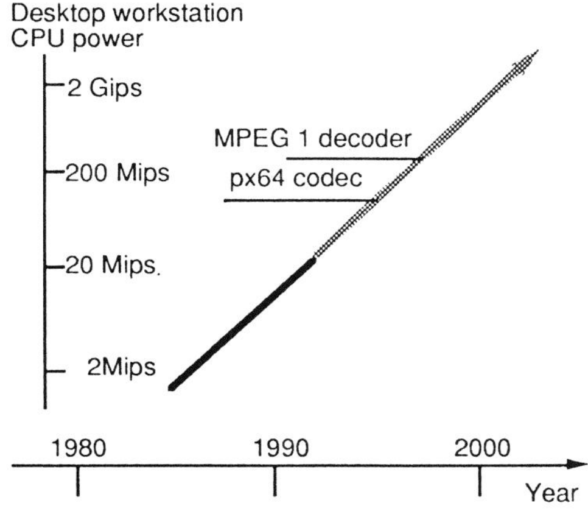

Fig. 8. Future development of desktop workstation CPU power.

5 Software-Only Codecs and Scalable Video

Today, a real-time MPEG-1 decoder is commercially available as a single board that plugs into a personal computer [17]. The corresponding MPEG-1 coder board has been announced for 1993. Special hardware to augment a workstation or PC is, however, only a temporary solution. We can extrapolate current technological trends to find that software-only codecs will soon be a reality. Gordon Bell has observed that the price of a computer of given physical size does not substantially change over time; however, its CPU power increases by a factor of 10 every 5 years [18]. "Bell's Law" is shown in Figure 8 for a desktop workstation. Today, our MPEG-1 software decoder runs on a Sun SPARC IPX workstation (a 28.5 Mips RISC machine) at 1/10 real time. Soon, the CPU power of a desktop workstation will be sufficient to run this program in real-time. Real-time encoding and decoding according to H.261 will be possible even earlier. Ten years from now, in the year 2002, our typical desktop multimedia workstation is expected to execute more than 1 billion RISC instructions per second. Main memory of more than 1 GByte could be loaded into the machine, which would allow storage of more than an hour of compressed motion video in RAM.

When integrating motion video into an open computer system with a software-only codec, coding and decoding algorithms need extra flexibility to cope with the varying computation, transmission, and display resources of the system. This extra flexibility today is commonly referred to as "scalability." To my knowledge, the term "scalable video" was coined 4-5 years ago by Andy Lippman at MIT, reminiscent of "scalable fonts." Scalability includes three issues:

1. *Scalable image size.* In a window system, the user wants to be able to resize the video frame flexibly. Of course, a large video window can display more detail than a small window. A naive solution would simply decode the image with all detail available, and then filter and subsample it to the desirable size. This strategy, however, is wasteful. Rather, we only want to read, transmit, and decode that portion of the information that is required to display the image at the desired size with satisfactory resolution.
2. *Partial decodability.* When transmitting video over networks operating in asynchronous transfer mode (ATM), the effective channel capacity is not known in advance. Rather, the video transmission is competing with other processes. As a consequence, the decoder has to be able to decode and display a picture from partial information. With network overload, the picture quality should degrade gracefully.
3. *Computation-limited coding and decoding.* In a multitasking environment, there are several processes competing for the computational resources of the same workstation. Similar to the unknown transmission bandwidth on ATM networks, there is an unknown computational bandwidth that affects both coding and decoding. This issue becomes even more severe in multipoint videoconferencing situations, where multiple bitstreams have to be decoded simultaneously. Moreover, we might want to decode the same bit-stream with processors of different power. Even low-end workstations should be able to decode a given motion video bit-stream, even though picture quality might be reduced compared to high-end workstations.

The scalability requirements listed above are quite different from those of the classical telecommunication situation, where there are well-defined source and display formats, a fixed transmission bit-rate, and coders and decoders which are digital circuits designed and optimized for their specific tasks. Relatively little attention has been paid to scalable video in the past. The CCITT H.261 video compression standard has no scalability at all. Even if only a few bits cannot be decoded, it might take several seconds until the picture recovers. MPEG-1 is somewhat scalable. If the channel or the decoder cannot keep up with the full bit-stream, we can leave out B-pictures without harm for other pictures. Unfortunately, B-pictures typically constitute the smaller part of the entire data. MPEG-1 has no mechanism for spatial scalability, i.e., pictures always have to be decoded to full resolution. MPEG-2 has included scalability in its requirements, however, it will probably only apply to the range between an embedded MPEG-1 bit-stream and the full MPEG-2 format. A truly scalable video code would support graceful degradation all the way down to zero.

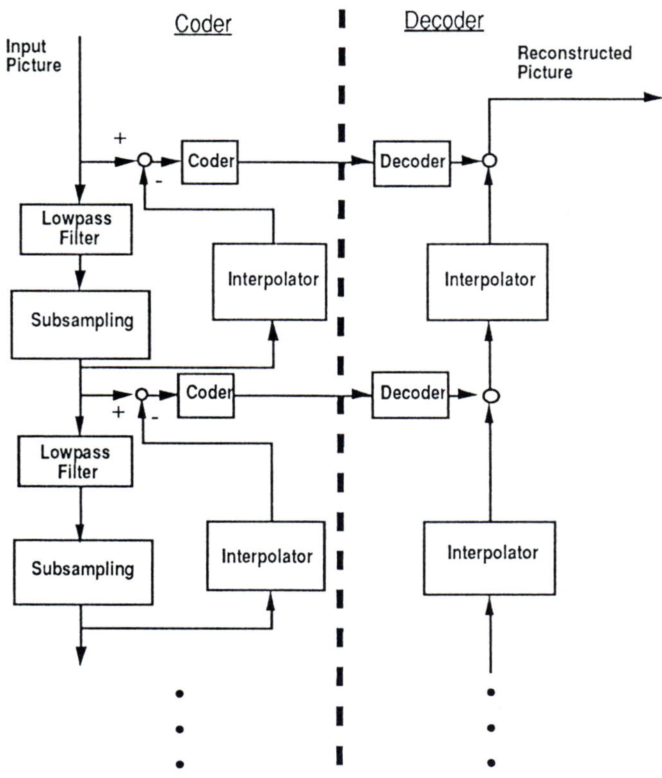

Fig. 9. block diagram of a resolution pyramid codec

Resolution pyramids, as illustrated in Figures 9 and 10, are a straightforward approach, and yet very suitable for scalable video applications. The full resolution input picture is filtered and subsampled several times. The interpolation error between levels is then encoded and transmitted. At the decoder, the image is interpolated several times, and the decoded interpolation error is added at the appropriate level of the pyramid. The resolution pyramid adds some redundancy initially, since there are more interpolation error samples to be transmitted then there are samples in the input picture. This extra redundancy has to be reduced in the interpolation error coders. For a subsampling of 4:1 (2:1 horizontally and vertically), as shown in Figure 10, the redundancy is bounded above by the geometric series $1 + \frac{1}{4} + \frac{1}{16} + \frac{1}{64} + \ldots = \frac{4}{3}$. Since the correlation between the signals of the individual pyramid levels is very small, independent encoding is justified.

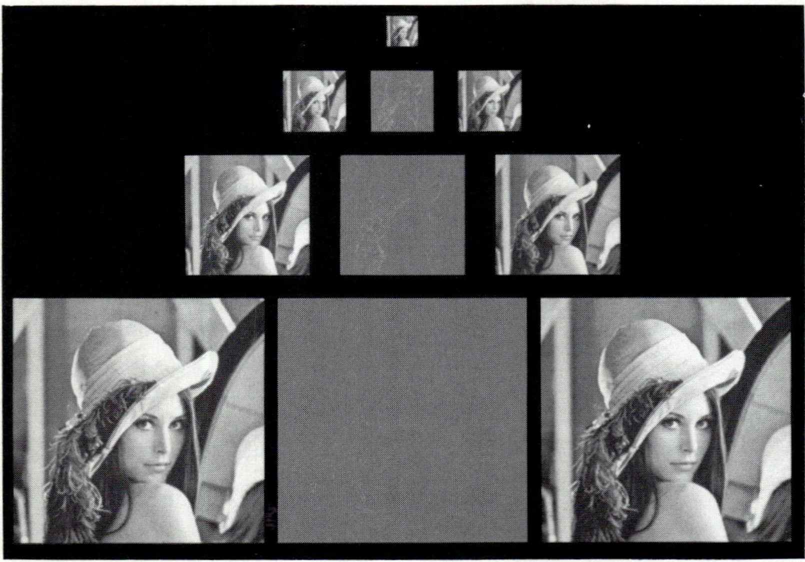

Fig. 10. Resolution pyramid. Filtered and subsampled images are shown on the left; the interpolated images are shown on the right. The middle stack shows the interpolation error pyramid to be encoded (from [21]).

It is also possible to decompose images into resolution pyramids without increasing the number of samples. This can be accomplished using the Discrete Wavelet Transform. Excellent compression results with this approach are reported for example in [9]. It is hard to combine these spatial wavelet decompositions with nonlinear techniques such as motion compensation, while this is straightforward with resolution pyramids [19].

A spatiotemporal resolution pyramid is shown in Figure 11. At the coder, every other frame is filtered and subsampled by 2:1 horizontally and vertically to form a sequence of reduced frame rate and size. This process is repeated to form another sequence that is subsampled 4:1 in each direction, and so on. Interpolation is carried out temporally with motion compensation, and the interpolation error is encoded. Then, each frame is spatially interpolated to the next resolution level, and again the interpolation error is encoded. This concept was originally proposed in [19]. As the geometric series $(1 + \frac{1}{8} + \frac{1}{64} + \frac{1}{512} + \ldots)$ converges to $\frac{8}{7}$, only very little redundancy is introduced by the pyramid decomposition.

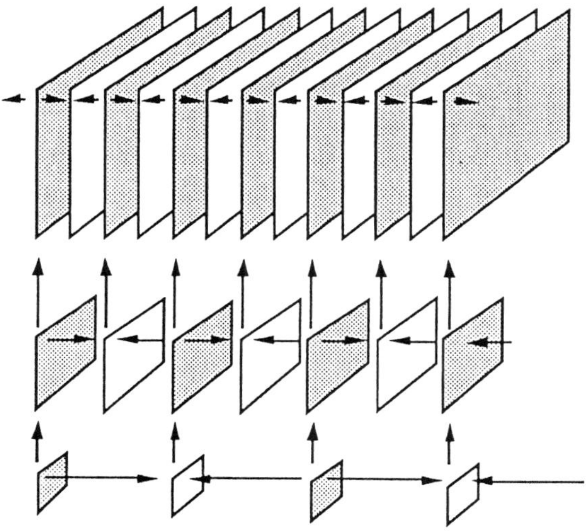

Fig. 11. Spatiotemporal resolution pyramid (from [21]).

Since the resolution pyramid decomposition is not unique for a given decoder, there is freedom to build coding schemes with varying degrees of asymmetry. For distribution applications, motion video is encoded once, but decoded many times. Therefore, the decoder should be as simple as possible, while the coder can be complex. The pyramid shown in Figure 10 uses an asymmetric subsampling filter/interpolator pair [21]. The interpolation requires about 1/6 of the operations compared to the lowpass filtering for subsampling. In addition to the pyramid decomposition/interpolation, displacement estimation lends itself naturally to building an asymmetric codec. Displacement estimation is carried out at the coder, and the displacement vectors are transmitted and used at the decoder. Therefore, motion estimation is not required at the decoder.

6 Delay Issues

For telephone conversations, round-trip delays of more than 250 ms are quite disturbing and limit the spontaneous interaction between the participants. For videoconferencing, similar numbers apply. Low bit-rate interframe coding methods introduce delay, since they exploit the dependency between successive frames, lower the frame rate, and buffer the spatial and temporal variations in information contents of the motion video. In general, low bit-rate implies long coding/decoding delay. If the picture round-trip delay is unacceptably large, it is usually better to sacrifice lip-synchonization and obtain a shorter delay for speech. Note that coder and decoder delays have to add up to a constant time interval, while the delay introduced by each of the buffers varies in a complementary fashion.

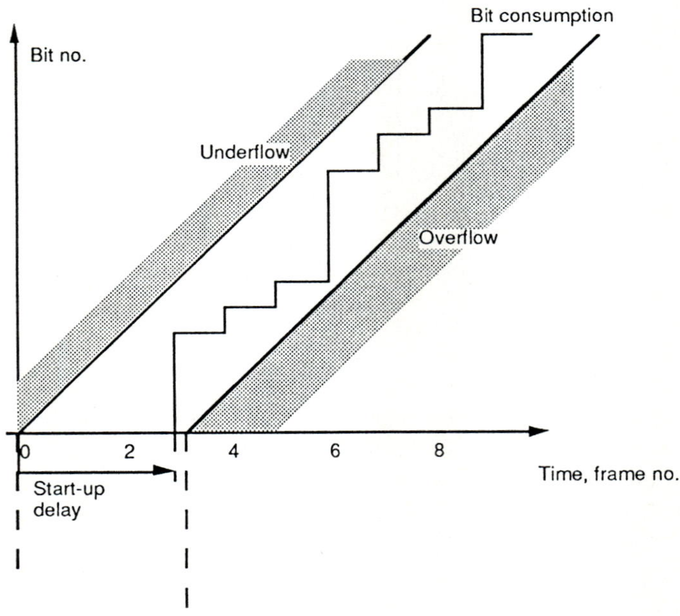

Fig. 12. Decoder buffer operation.

For storage of interactive video, the decoding delay should be as short as possible. The shorter the delay, the more immediate the interaction is with the video signal. A typical decoder buffer operation is shown in Figure 12. We assume that bits are provided by a storage medium at a constant rate, corresponding to the underflow limit in Figure 12. The bit consumption of the decoder varies. Some pictures require a large amount of bits, while for others only a small amount is required. This is due to variations in picture contents and the various encoding modes used for different frames, as e.g., I-pictures, P-pictures, and B-pictures in MPEG. The buffer has limited capacity; thus an overflow results if the delay between bit supply and consumption were to exceed a maximum. When accessing a new video sequence, the start-up delay will be close to the maximum value, since the first picture has to be encoded without reference to other frames. It is not a viable strategy to fill the decoder buffer to some level close to its maximum and then start decoding and displaying the first frame. With this strategy, additional headroom is required to prevent overflow and underflow, leading to unnecessary delays. Instead, the video bit stream should contain time stamp information at each potential entry point, which would determine the precise start-up delay of the decoder buffer. It turns out that with time stamping, the decoder buffer need be precisely half the size as without it. Note that MPEG-1 uses time-stamping as described to reduce the decoder buffer delay.

7 Conclusions

Fully digital integration of motion video offers many advantages over the coupling of conventional analog video technology with computers. I have discussed a variety of problems to be overcome for such an integration. The bit-rate for an uncompressed digitized video signal is too high to fit on current storage devices or to pass through local area networks, thus necessitating video compression. Techniques standardized to date, such as CCITT H.261 or MPEG-1, are not ideally suited for motion video integration into computer systems, since they lack scalability. Scalability should include image size scalability, partial bit-stream decodability, and computation-limited coding and decoding. Resolution-pyramids are a straightforward approach to build a scalable video codec. This concept can be extended to a 3D spatiotemporal resolution pyramid with motion compensation. Finally, we have discussed delay problems that arise with interframe coding both for videoconferencing and for stored video. Time-stamping is essential to minimize the decoding delay for stored video.

As I have argued in section 5, real-time video codecs can be simply software for desktop computers a few years from now. The lack of suitable standards for scalable video might require several multimedia computer manufacturers to provide their own proprietary video compression schemes. While this would be disastrous in a world of hardware codecs, it should ultimately not be a problem with software codecs. Chances are that future multimedia computers will be able to decode several proprietary formats in addition to MPEG and the CCITT px64 standards.

References

1. J. Nielsen, "Hypertext and Hypermedia," San Diego: Academic Press, 1990.
2. S. Brand, "The Media Lab: Inventing the Future at MIT," Viking Penguin, 1987.
3. I. Greif (ed.), "Computer-supported cooperative work: a book of readings," San Mateo: Morgan Kaufman Publishers, 1988.
4. H. Delpho, "Der Multimediamarkt in West Europa und USA," in Proc. Telematica, Multimedia 2000, Stuttgart, Germany, Sept./Oct. 1992.
5. "Encoding parameters of digital television for studios," CCIR Recommendation 601, 1982.
6. N. S. Jayant and P. Noll, "Digital Coding of Waveforms," Englewood Cliffs, NJ: Prentice-Hall, 1984.
7. A. N. Netravali and B. G. Haskell, "Digital Pictures - Representation and Compression," Plenum Press, New York, London, 1988.
8. J. R. Jain and A. K. Jain, "Displacement measurement and its application to interframe image coding," IEEE Transactions on Communications, vol. 29, no. 12, pp. 1799 - 1809, Dec. 1981.
9. T. Senoo, B. Girod, "Vector Quantization for Entropy Coding of Image Subbands," IEEE Transactions on Image Processing, vol. 1, no. 3, October 1993.
10. O. Rioul and M. Vetterli, "Wavelets and Signal Processing," IEEE Signal Processing Magazine, vol. , pp. 14 - 38, October 1991.
11. A. E. Jacquin, "Image Coding Based on a Fractal Theory of Iterated Contractive Image Transformations," IEEE Trans. on Image Processing, vol. 1, no. 1, pp. 18 - 30, January 1992.
12. R. Forchheimer and T. Kronander, "Image Coding - From Waveforms to Animation," IEEE Transactions on Acoustics, Speech, and Signal Processing, vol. vol. 37, no. no. 12, pp. 2008 - 2023, December 1989.
13. "Coding of moving pictures and associated audio," standard ISO 11172, 1991
14. D. LeGall, "MPEG: A Video Compression Standard for Multimedia Applications," Communications of the ACM, vol. 34, no. 4, pp. 46 - 58, April 1991.
15. B. Girod, "Motion-compensating prediction with fractional-pel accuracy," IEEE Transactions on Communications, to appear April 1993.
16. "Video codec for audio visual services at px64 kbit/s," CCIR Recommendation H.261, CDM XV-R-37-E, August 1990.
17. B. Girod, D. LeGall, H. G. Musmann, G. Wallace, "Data Compression for Multimedia Systems," panel presentation at Siggraph '92, Chicago, IL, July 1992.
18. C. G. Bell, "Toward a History of (Personal) Workstations," in A. Goldberg (ed.), "A History of Personal Workstations," New York, ACM Press, pp. 1 - 50, 1988.
19. K. M. Uz, M. Vetterli, and D. J. LeGall, "Interpolative Multiresolution Coding of Advanced Television with Compatible Subchannels," IEEE Transactions on Circuits and Systems for Video Technology, vol. 1, no. 1, pp. 86 - 99, March 1991.
20. Ming Liou, "Overview of the px64 kbit/s Video Coding Standard," Communications of the ACM, vol. 34, no. 4, pp. 59 - 63, April 1991.
21. B. Girod, "Scalable Video for Multimedia Workstations," Computers and Graphics, to appear in vol. 17, no. 3, 1993.

A Modeling / Programming Framework for Large Media-Integrated Applications

Max Mühlhäuser
Computer Science Dept., Institute for Telematics, Telecooperation Group
University of Karlsruhe, D-76128 Karlsruhe, Germany
max@tk.telematik.informatik.uni-karlsruhe.de

1 Introduction

Most present multimedia applications represent selfcontained off-the-shelf tools for specific tasks. We believe that in order for multimedia technology to gain widespread use, *media-integrated* applications must be emphasized; such applications integrate customized multimedia use with 'conventional' applications, using enterprise workflow models as the embracing concept.

Today, however, the development of large and cooperative media-integrated applications is a painful and cumbersome crafting task, due to the lack of an adequate software technology. As a consequence, we propose the development of a more adequate software technology which we coin as the move from object-oriented to *items-oriented* programming. Cooperative media-integrated applications will rapidly gain importance in the future for the following three reasons.

Cooperation trend: multimedia base technology evolves rapidly and is marked by a tight integration of three large market segments: consumer electronics, information technology, and telecommunications. Example elements of this base technology include ATM switches and networks, 'multimedia-proof' communication protocols (ST2, XTP, ec.) and storage technology (CD-ROM extensions, document architectures, databases), media servers in distributed systems, compression standards like JPEG and MPEG, and videophone standards like the H.200-series. Many existing multimedia *applications*, however, represent selfcontained off-the-shelf tools for very specific tasks ('authoring' systems for multimedia presentations, videoconferencing tools, etc.).

This is in drastic contrast to the *integration* trend which marks many software application domains, such as Computer-Integrated Manufacturing and Engineering (CIM, CIE), and office automation. Such integration, in turn, is viewed as the base for better *cooperation* support in an organization; cooperation, here, has two facets:

- *Workflow-type cooperation:* organizations try to make better use of their large enterprise networks by integrating their formerly isolated application packages; thereby, outputs of packages are fed into other ones in an intelligent way, packages mutually call one another, and, most important, superimposed workflow management software manages and traces the flow of work in the organization.

- *CSCW-type cooperation:* computer-supported cooperative work -CSCW-, together with workflow management, is supposed to lead to enhanced cooperation of all parts of an enterprise (supply chain, production process, etc.); with CSCW-type cooperation, the focus is on the *humans* involved.

Media integration demand: in the context of this integration / cooperation trend, multimedia is no more an end in itself, but a requirement. Workflow-type cooperation requires *entire* activity records and documents to be computerized (traditional database applications kept only short, abstract descriptions: database records). This leads to the use of multimedia objects such as scanned images, digitized audio annotations, video and audio conference recordings, summarized as *persistent media*. CSCW-type cooperation, on the other hand, requires *transient* media to be captured, transmitted and presented in real time (video / audio conferencing, application sharing, etc.).

Software technology requirement: A look at current software technology shows that traditional software development tools are totally inadequate for large distributed applications. E.g., the majority of CASE environments focus on sequential software intended to run on a single computer. As to distributed applications, there is a strong focus on client/server- (and, along with this, RPC-) based techniques; strict client/server-structures, however, do not match very well with the complex, irregular organizational structures of an enterprise. And the integration of distributed application engineering with multimedia and cooperation support (in both facets, workflow and CSCW) is hardly approached at all.

To summarize, we see a heavy need for a new era in software technology, enabling effective production of

- large and distributed
- media-integrated
- cooperative (workflow-type and CSCW-type)

application software. We want to use the term **CMA** (cooperative media-integrated applications) in the remainder to denote this type of application. In the following, we will recall major lessions which we learned in predecessor projects and describe the embedding of our work in the current project context. We will then sketch major aspects of an adequate framework for the development of CMAs.

2 Background

2.1 Experiences and Requirements

For the proposed framework, we draw from the experience gained in several predecessor projects, undertaken jointly with other universities and industrial research groups. Three of these projects are to be mentioned here.

Project Docase [GZH90,MGH93] lead to a modeling / programming framework for large (non-multimedia) distributed applications. The key lessons learned were as follows:

- Distributed object-oriented programming languages form an excellent basis for the development of large distributed applications. In particular, they exhibit three features which we summarize as *distribution transparency*:
  - such languages provide for location independent operation ('method') invocation (i.e., local and remote 'procedure' calls are semantically equivalent).
  - since design and implementation usually yield a large number of *small* objects, decisions about the distribution of these objects over a target network can be deferred to installation time; in particular, distribution aspects do not have to be taken into account during design.
  - if object migration is supported, distribution decisions can even be altered at runtime.
- Adequate modeling and design support is crucial for the successful development of large object-oriented programs: a huge number of objects have to be handled on the implementation level, making object-oriented programs even less managable than conventional ones. Docase supports modeling on the base of socalled "object categories", a concept that will be explained and expanded in the context of the new framework proposed in this paper.
- For mission-critical software, lots of so-called "operational" aspects need attention, such as authorization, authenication, reliability, and accounting. With current software engineeering techniques, all these aspects are mangled into the mainstream application code. Therefore, a new modularization concept was developed, called 'program superimposition', extending work described in [Kat93]. In chapter 3, we will motivate the application of this concept in the context of the proposed new framework.

In the Nestor project [MüS92], we developed services and tools for the development of cooperative media-integrated *courseware* (computer-based teaching or instruction material). On one hand, Nestor lead to a series of different multimedia and CSCW tools, such as a software video codec, a tool for recording Xwindow output to a file for further processing, and a tool which augments Xwindow applications for cooperative use. On the other hand, applying these tools in computer aided instruction made us aware of the need for a much more integrative, customizable approach to courseware (and software) construction. In this respect, we learned the following lessons from Nestor:

- the marriage of object-oriented concepts and hypertext leads to an appealing and powerful new concept
- support for *distributed* multimedia aspects is essential; distribution *transparency* is particularly important, but needs substantial additions to the known approaches mentioned above (i.e., distributed object-oriented techniques)
- while applications can be tranparently augmented for a primitive level of cooperation support, real "cooperation awareness" needs a substantial development effort; at present, *generic* CSCW programming tools hardly exist.

The third predecessor project, DIRECT, represents a 'hand-crafted' sample CMA which served for gathering requirements about the framework proposed in chapter 3. DIRECT supports physically distributed research or engineering teams with a set of integrated cooperation and task management tools. It is centered around the "issue-based design" metaphor for organizing ill-structured problems, originally described in [Pot89]. Direct showed that

- an integrated CMA can support the users much better than a set of isolated tools
- such a CMA can be partly made up from pre-built components, provided the components are highly customizable (programmable)
- workflows and human cooperation, as supported by a CMA, are highly interrelated; a common modeling concept for both is desirable.

2.2 Project Organization

The work described in chapter 3 is embedded into the B.I.G. embracing project whose major sponsor is Digital Equipment:

B stands for Berkom, a stretegic project in Germany, which runs under the auspices of the research and development spin-off of the german PTT, DTBerkom Several multimedia services and tool suites are built as part of the project. Digital is one of the major industrial partners in the project, our group is invoved in the development of multimedia collaboration (MMC) and multimedia mail (MMM) tool suites [ADH93].

I stands for Items, the project in which the CMA development framework is developed by our group. This part is described in more detail in the following section.

G stands for 'Gigaswitch', a new switching technology developed by Digital with an aggregate throughput of several Gigabits per second. Gigaswitch connects FDDI-based computers, but in contrast to standard FDDI, a star topology connects the FDDI stations point-to-point, so that the full FDDI speed can be exploited by every station. due to the use of dedicated point-to-point links, Gigaswitch networks can assure quality of service parameters that make them much more suitable for multimedia communication than standard FDDI. Future members of the Gigaswitch familiy are supposed to assure transition to ATM.

In summary, the B and G parts of the BIG project allow our Items activities to be embedded into a large testbed which relates our work to many national and international activities, and which provides dedicated and multimedia-proof high-speed connectivity; Berkom, in addition, provides tools and software pieces which we can use to evaluate our integration concepts.

3 Proposed Framework

3.1 Overview, Item-Oriented Programming

This chapter is devoted to the description of a framework for the development of CMAs. The project and development environment are called 'Items', referring to the idea of 'item-oriented programming'. This term is meant to show that on one hand, we use object-oriented programming as our basis, but on the other hand, we extend the functionality of objects for better support of cooperation and multimedia aspects (the term item can be understood as the acronym for '*i*conic *te*lecooperating *m*ultimedia object)

Since we want to give an idea about the overall Items system, some details will have to be related to more in-depth papers mentioned in the references. Some parts of items represent revised and extended versions of modules and concepts developed in the predecessor projects mentioned. The Items system is still under construction since the project is in a relatively early stage. In particular, the system still consists of loosely coupled parts whose integration has not been achieved yet. The experiences gained in predecessor projects, however, makes us confident that most of the serious problems have been resolved and that the concepts described in the remainder represent a feasible approach.

We will first give a coarse view of the overall Items architecture and the major tool-building-tool which we are using (section 3.1). In section 3.3, we will concentrate on the item-oriented design and programming model. Thereby, we will give a short overview of the top-level so-called 'item categories' available. In sections 3.4 through 3.7, we will describe the functionality of some of these categories in more detail, concentrating on the following aspects for brevity: an introduction to our support for distributed object-oriented programming in general (very coarsely discussed), support for distributed multimedia, support for workflow-type and CSCW-type cooperation, and support for re-usable hypertext structures.

3.2 Items System Architecture

The Items system represents a whole software engineering environment with several modeling, programming and monitoring tools, code management support, and integration facilities on the data, tool, and UI layers. Fig. 3.1 concentrates on those components of the Items system which are crucial for the design and execution of item-oriented CMAs.

The most important tool is called *VIP* (visual item-oriented program design tool). VIP accompanies the programmers throughout the design and implementation phases. It integrates both the graphical and the textual programming metaphor. VIP supports graphical programming of the coarse and fine grained design, including dynamic aspects. Code is automatically generated from design. There is no virtual boundary between design and implementation; instead, textual programming of software modules can be carried out in the context of the graphical entities managed by VIP. Thus, a seamless integration of design and programming, of visual and textual program development is supported. The sections below will describe the elements of graphical programming ('item categories').

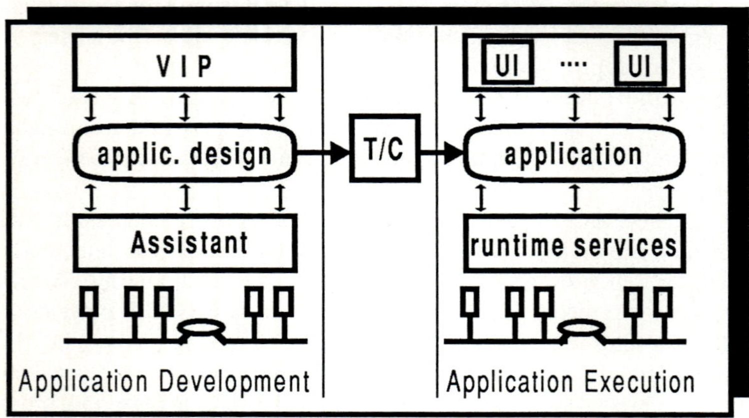

Fig. 3.1. Core tools and services of the Items system

VIP is built using a very generic tool-biulding-tool developed in our group, called ODE. ODE (object-oriented design editor) was used to build many different graphical tools and interfaces in the past. It is based on a very flexible object model that can be customized to the needs of the tool under construction. For customization of ODE, a Lisp dialect is used; C and C++ routines can be linked into the code. Different graph layout algorithms are attached to ODE via a special layout subsystem called LAMA. Currently, ODE is extended for use in distributed software engineering environments and for cooperation with heterougeneous programming tools.

Apart from VIP; the so-called *Items Design Assistant* has to be mentioned. The development of this assistant stems from the fact that many design notations (graphical, textual-language-based, or else) are associated with a design *method,* i.e with strategies and rules to follow during design. Most design *tools,* however, hardly support the respective method; this is especially true for methods which are not totally 'formal', because their respective methods cannot be expressed in the context of the design notation. The Items Design Assistant uses a separate formal language to describe an informally given development method, mapping it to building blocks and operations of the design methods, to artifacts of the application under development, and -most important - to different types of artifacts which represent the reasoning about the design (steps, issues, arguments, etc.). The concept of a Design Assistant has been successfully used in the Docase project already (cf. [MGH93]).

As fig. 3.1 indicates, an application is transformed into executable code by special transformation / compilation tools. Thereby, the graphical information is transformed into source code and interleaved with the textual program parts. This leads to purely textual source code which is compiled. The current version of Items supports a distributed version of C++ (called DC++) which was developed at our Institute. We intend to support a more elegant distributed object-oriented programming in the future, a successor of the DOWL language developed in our group [Ach91]. DOWL is a strongly typed multiple-inheritance language which supports object migration even for objects which are in execution. The language currently supported, DC++, is not as elegant (due to the ancestors, C and C++), but powerful enough to reach distribution transparency in the context of Items.

At runtime, an item-oriented CMA relies on a number of sophisticated runtime services, partly described below. In particular, we will describe the service which provides distribution transparency in the presence of multimedia objects. Fig. 3.1 also indicates the decoupling of the core of item-oriented applications from their user interface part, which is described further below, too.

3.3 Item Categories

Rationale: So-called *class libraries* have become a common approach in the object-oriented community. In analogy to 'function libraries' of conventional languages, such class libraries contain the definitions of pre-built 'kinds of objects' (called 'classes' or 'types', depending on the programming language) which together represent the core functionality of a certain problem domain. E.g., 'Interviews' is a very well-known C++ class library for the programming of window-based graphical interfaces, making live much easier than with plain Xwindow programming. Two major problems restrict the value of class libraries:

- When an application programmer uses a class library, he will usually have difficulties to learn the syntax and semantics of the pre-defined object classes. He will mostly have to depend on manuals and on the level of checking a compiler can provide; the compiler, however, will 'understand' little of the semantics of the object classes and nothing about the semantics of the way in which they are to be used in an application - most checking will be on the syntactic level.
- Large applications, CMAs in particular, will exploit many different facets and aspects of functionality. A programmer will therefore want to use several different class libraries. However, it is a common experience in large software projects that only a very small number of different libraries or APIs can be integrated with a single application program, due to the necessary effort to understand the different 'mind sets', 'models', and ways of usage associated with pre-built libraries or APIs.

In the items project, we try to overcome these problems by using the so-called 'category approach'. Categories are pre-built object classes in the first place, but their semantics are 'understood' by the programming tools and they cover the complete software development, not only a small domain like graphical interface programming.

For further discussion, we refer to fig. 3.2. The somewhat 'condensed' layout in this figure shows a tree with a root (parent node, called 'item') and two levels of child nodes (first level: shapes only, no icons; second level: shapes *and* icons); at one point, the third level is included as well (child nodes of 'interactor').

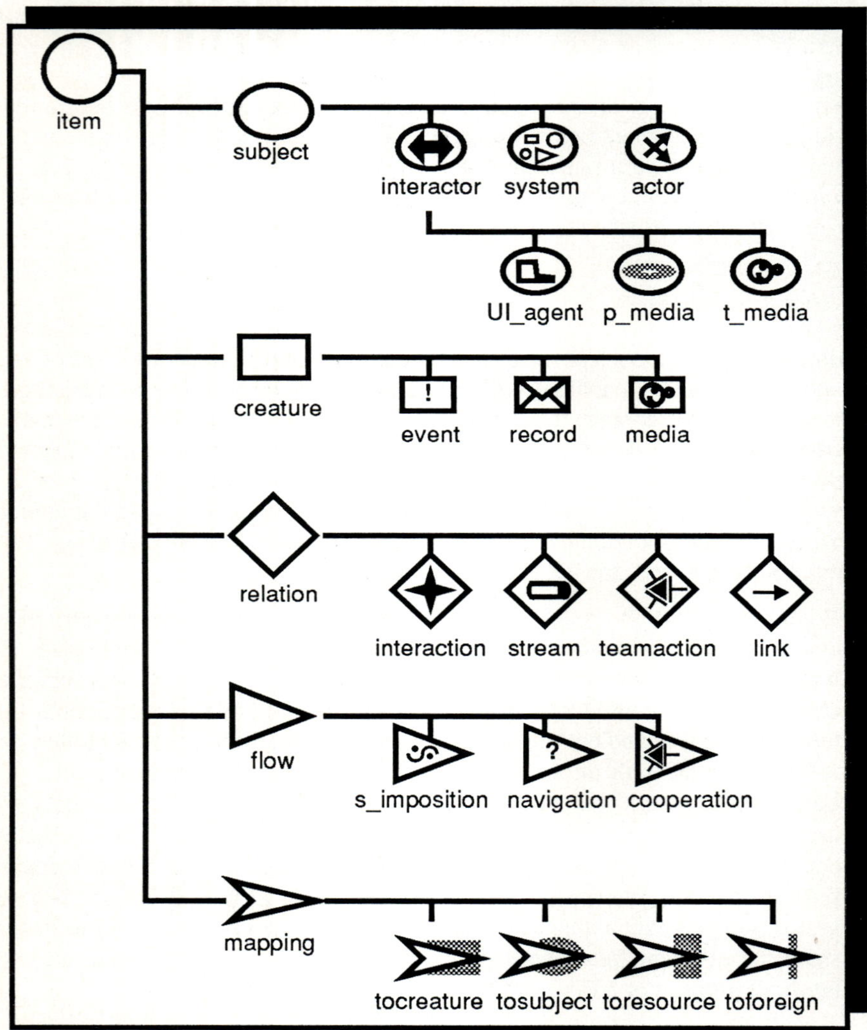

Fig. 3-2 Item Categories

The main functionality of item categories can now be explained more precisely; thereby, the differences to the common 'class libraries' should become obvious:

- A whole item-oriented CMA is made up of 'items': every class definition used in an application must be derived from one (or several) of the categories shown in fig. 3.2. Of course, every object (or item, to be more precise) in an application must in turn be an *instance* of such a class definition.
- The first level of categories below root (subject, creature, relation, flow, and mapping) represents 'orthogonal' 'meta' categories. 'Orthogonal' means that any class definition must be derived from *exactly one* of these five top-level categories (the items in an application can thus be divided into five disjunct sets). 'Meta' means that instances cannot be directly created from one of these categories, but only from their children and further descendants (sub-classes).
- The VIP graphical/textual program development tool offers sophisticated support to the software engineers as they develop an item-oriented CMA. Starting from the palette of item meta-categories, the tool allows to select an actual category of choice, to create or modify subtypes of this category (class-based view), to define instances of a class or to redefine the class from which they are derived (instance view), or to reason about various dynamic relationships between classes or instances (scenario view). Since VIP 'knows' the semantics of the categories, it guides the user as he specifies parts, relationships and behaviour of a class and as he interconnects items in the design.
- The Items Assistant can be used to arrange the VIP-based micro-level design operations (adding or modification of classes or instances) into macro-level steps according to an embracing design method and general design rules.

In the remainder of this section, we will give an overview of the item categories, to the level of detail depicted in fig. 3.2 (note that further sub-categories exist):

Subject. The subject meta-category represents the entities that make up the backbone 'configuration' of an application. An initial configuration of subjects must be defined within any application; subjects can be added, removed, or migrated between nodes only by means of explicit 'configuration changes'. In contrast to 'creatures', subjects typically have threads of control of their own, i.e. they can act asynchronously and in parallel to other items. The following major subcategories of 'subject' exist:

- *interactor:* this category provides interfaces to human-perceivable information representations; such information is supposed to come from or go to parts of the system which are external to the applications, such as multimedia devices or archives, and multimedia user interfaces. Three sub-categories of interactors are depicted in fig. 3.2:
  - *UI_agent:* this category plays an emportant role for ensuring high portablity of item-oriented applications. It is motivated by the experiences with window-based graphical user interfaces (GUIs) based on common windowing systems such as Motif or Windows. These systems usually offer a very low level interface between the core application and the GUI: the 'look and feel' has to be described in terms of geometric data, and many window-system

specific details have to be programmed (he GUI server code itself cannot be changed usually). This problem lead to the development of several systems which support the use of several GUIs transparently. These approaches encapsulate differences between different windowing systems, making applications more portable.
The UI_agent category in items goes one step further: it encapsulates differences between UIs that are based on different media and metaphors (MUIs). UI_agents come with a skeletal, high-level “application-to-UI protocol” (where, e.g. the window-based concept "menu" is replaced by the more abstract concept "selection", "scope-change" replaces "zoom/pan", etc.) and with implementations for different MUI types (first version: window-based and speech-enahnced). Both the protocol and the MUIs can be customized to accomodate specific application needs and further MUI types.

- *p_media:* ‘permanent’ multimedia archives are encapsulated by this category, covering the range from simple file store to document storage servers, multimedia kiosks, and multimedia databases. The interface to a p_media item may include queries and discrete and continuous media storage/ retrieval. The ‘subject’ nature of p_media allows it to model, e.g., asynchonous (‘overnight’) delivery of information.
- *t_media:* the ‘transient’ t_media items encapsulate capturing and presentation devices such as cameras, microphones, displays, scanners, etc. Asynchronous behaviour, here, may occur from the possibility for the user to switch the device on or off or to carry out other local operations which the computer can become aware of. Special synchronization support for multple media is given according to the concept described in [BHL92].

- *system:* the system category compensates one of the lacks of conventional object-oriented systems: while such systems provide an excellent means for modelling ‘kind of’ relations by inheritence, they support ‘part of’ relations only marginally, usually by providing an ‘aggregate’ concept. ‘System’ items represent the major concept for hierarchical (and overlapping) decomposition of an application configuration. They enhance the ‘part of’ concept considerably: e.g., a system can offer an interface to the external items which completely hides the internal structure and contents. The role-resolution concept (described further below) can be used for mapping the ‘external’ interface to the content items of a system. Based on its own thread, a system controls its internal configuration (number and types of configurable items, their interconnection via ‘relation’ items, etc.) as well as the role-resolution.
- *actors*: very similar to the ‘active object’ concept available in some object-oriented systems, actors may contain several (light-weigth) threads of their own for which they manage concurrency and synchronization; actors dispatch incoming requests autonomously.

Creature. The term ‘creature’ indicates that items of this category are created at runtime. They are not considered part of the so-called ‘application configuration’.

Migration of 'creatures' can be determined autonomously by the 'object placement service' of the runtime system (unless explicitly forbidden by the programmer). Intuitively spoken, creatures model parts of an application which are created and destroyed 'in masses', such as mails, route slips which accompany parts in a production plant, or database records. Three sub-categories are relevant:

- *event:* this category models the classical 'software trap' concept and is used for asynchronous activation of subjects.
- *record:* on one hand, records represent the 'default' modeling for 'standard' objects which do not differ from the kinds of objects found in a conventional object-oriented system. On the other hand, the system support for migration, propagation and routing of records makes their 'journey' through a distributed system more efficient. Like media (see below), records are exchanged between subjects, either directly or via 'relations'.
- *media:* the media category provides the unique system model for all kinds of single media and multimedia data. Its interface includes a set of generic operations (display, create, edit, etc.) and a 'quality of service' concept. More details will be given in section 3.4.

Relation. With the 'system' category explained above, we compensated for deficiencies in the object-oriented 'part of' relation. The relation category now compensates for deficiencies in the object-oriented 'knows' relation. in object-oriented systems, one object 'knows' another one when it knows its unique identifier (typically, this identifier is stored in a so-called 'instance variable'). Any object may call operations of any other object it 'knows', thereby establishing a temporary communication relation. Thus, the communication relations between objects are 'hidden' in the application program and neither explicitly modeled nor easily tracked at runtime. For items, we introduce an explicit 'relation' category which can be used to model binary and n-ary 'communication paths'. The following four sub-categories add more functionality to this concept.

- *interaction:* this category provides so-called communication schedules as described in [ScG91]. They support multiparty relations and multi-stage communiction (several subsequent interrelated communications). The communicating subject items involved are described via roles (which are resolved at runtime).
- *stream:* in order to transport continuous media, 'streams' can be defined. Such streams make efficient use of the underlying transport system and do not provide direct access to the data transferred (these data have to be extracted via the interface of the 'media' category described above). Streams are also handled by the distributed runtime service described in 3.4
- *teamaction:* the concept for generic CSCW-type cooperation support (described in section 3.5 below) is founded on the idea that standard objects (more precisely: specific item categories such as media and record) can be extended to team-objects by adding a 'teamaction' context to their operation. See below for more details.

- *link:* this relation category adds basic hypertext functionality to the items model. Links are mainly used in the context of 'navigations' (see below and section 3.6). A link connects subjects cas its 'sources' and 'destinations'; the latter can be determined at instanciation time (static link) or at the time a 'navigation' traverses the link (computed link).

Flow. In contrast to relations and similar to subjects, flows contain threads of their own. A flow is a kind of 'global thread' which may traverse many different subjects; it is, however, long-lived and persistent (a flow may take on for months) and not bound to any particular subject. A flow is not 'hosted' in a particular network node and traverses node boundaries at will.

- *s_imposition:* as mentioned in chapter 2, the extended superimposition concept used in items represents a way of coping with the multitude of 'operational aspects' (accounting, security, reliability...) of large CMAs. The s_imposition category contains both a 'global thread' (in the context of which certain operational aspects have to be considered) *and* a description about how the operational aspects are to be intertwined with the 'global thread' (and with all the items called from there. This describtion uses parametrized code fragments and so-called 'filters' which determine the details of how the fragments have to be intertwined with other pieces of code (items, parts therein, parameter settings etc.), based on a kind of formal semantics. We will not describe this fundamental concept in more detail since it is not central to the problems of cooperation and multimedia; rather, we point to a fundamental article about program superimposition and to our own work in this respect [Kat93, Heu90].
- *cooperation:* this common modelling concept for both workflow-type and CSCW-type cooperation will be described in 3.5
- *navigation:* a navigation can be seen as a 'global thread' which carries a 'user' through a series of subjects and links. Apart from the classical understanding of 'hypertext navigation' which supports users in reading complex documents, navigation items may support individuals to carry out multiple activities in a coordinated way, e.g., during a software development process. As such, navigations complement the 'multi-user' cooperations with a 'single user' global thread. The navigation concept will be elaborated in 3.6.

Mapping. Much of the runtime flexibility of item-oriented CMAs is due to the four role-resolution concepts included, called mappings:

- *tocreature:* this mapping can be used if the determination of the specific creature used in an application involves a non-trivial selection at runtime. E.g., different creatures may play a certain creature_role at different times; in this case, the embracing program defines a 'creature_role', and the 'tocreate' mapping defines both the required properties and the process of determining the specific creatures to fulfil the role.
- *tosubject:* in analogy to the above, 'tosubject' defines how 'subject roles' are resolved. This category will usually be much more important than the above one, used in relations and flows in many ways.

- *toresource:* resources in items comprise humans, devices, nodes, and schedulable resources such as bandwidth and compute time (corresponding sub-categories exist). As to humans, the 'toresource' maps person roles (e.g., as used in cooperations) to individuals at runtime). Network nodes and schedulable resources are taken into account by the multimedia object service described in 3.5, by the 'object placement' service mentioned in 3.4, and by 'interactor' items.
- *toexternal:* CMAs will hardly ever be built from scratch. Apart from item-oriented software modules to be reused, 'legacy software' will have to be included. In order to connect such legacy software to an item-oriented CMA, we use a concept which conforms to the CORBA 'object request broker' standard issued by the 'OMG' standardization body (object management group).

3.4 Distributed Object-Oriented Programming

Since this paper concentrates on the cooperation and multimedia aspects of CMA programming, we want to mention the general aspects of support for large distributed programs in items only very briefly. During the above section, however, it should have become evident that the item-oriented programming concept covers all aspects of distributed programming, not just cooperation and multimedia in particular. This reflects our central goal to support *media-integrated* applications. In addition to the distributed object-oriented concept, which already provides an excellent ground for the development of large distributed programs, items provides particular support for substantially enhanced modeling and target customization.

Modeling is enhanced through the category concept which allows software engineers to structure their application design in a 'standardized' way; category-based designs can be better understood and more easily communicated to peer software engineers, managers and users. Relation categories and flows help to make the 'behaviour' of the system much more evident, superimpositions provide for modularization and re-use of 'operational' aspects, and systems support better decomposition.

Target customization means that the same application code can be used in different or evolving runtime environments. For this end, too, items provides serveral concepts: sophisticated role resolution is supported with the mapping categories; automatic dynamic object placement is carried out by a runtime service which automatically migrates creatures (and selected other items) according to a heuristics-based algorithm (which minimizes inter-node communication, cf. [Sch90]); superimposition, again, is important since it allows to superimpose different operational algorithms at different times or for different target environments.

3.5 Distributed Multimedia Object Service

As discussed earlier, distribution transparency is essential for development frameworks for large distributed programs in general. Thus, it has to be assured for item-oriented programming in particular. However, distribution transparency is particularly hard to maintain in the presence of multimedia information. e.g., fig. 3.3 depicts part of an application scenario which works with a multimedia 'stream' established between a p_media source and a two t_media sinks. The operation semantics behind this scenario might be "play video x on the displays of persons y and z". Distribution transparency, in this context, means that the programmer need not care about the location of the video and the displays, neither about the available network bandwidths, storage formats, supported compression formats etc.

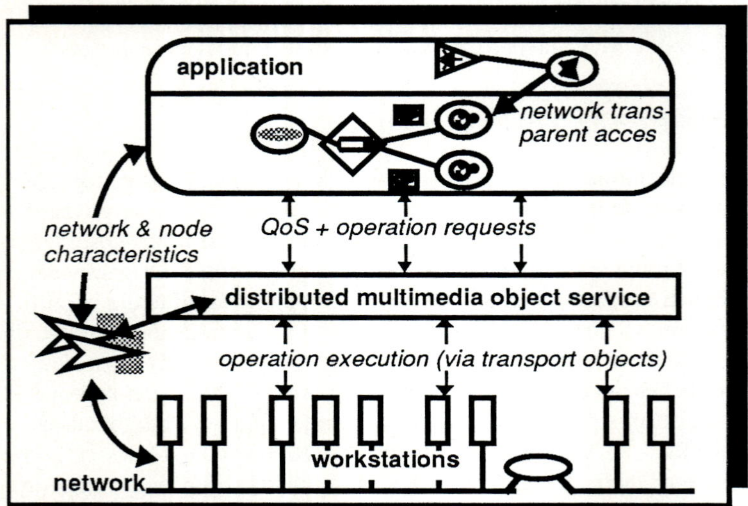

Fig. 3.3: Distribution Transparency for Multimedia Objects

To this end, we developed a distributed multimedia object service called MODE [Bla92]. Mode is based on descriptions of the 'environment' of an application (networks and workstation characteristics), given as 'toresource' mappings. It uses the item-oriented multimedia object model and therefore 'understands' the quality of service requirements and the operation calls issued by an application.

MODE is based on internal models of 'presentation objects' (cf. t_media and p_media items), 'information objects' (cf. media items), and 'transport objects' (optimized for transport in a network, invisible to the item-oriented program). In our example, the 'environment information' and the source and sink 'presentation' objects are used for an optimization at runtime.

Based on a 'decision tree', this optimization yields a so-called 'path' at runtime, composed of (source/sink) presentation objects and of transport objects (in a different example, 'information objects' could be included as well). This path represents the sequence of media transformations, transports, and manipulations which alltogether carry out the required operation under the given QoS constraints. In the example, MODE might find out that there is a low-bspeed bridge between source and destination requiring video compression, and that next to the users' workstations there is a station which can carry out decompression in hardware.

3.6 Cooperation Support

The cooperation support is centered around the item categories 'teamaction' and 'cooperation', based on predecessor work described in [Rüd91].

The *cooperation* category describes 'global threads' of parallel and sequential activities with a mix of flow-oriented and rule-based techniques. A partial, flow-oriented set of activities can be described as a 'task'. Such a task is described as a set of parallel and sequential activities, each of which is guarded by activation conditions and by required results which mark successful completion. Tasks can be assembled into cooperations based on a set of ordering rules (this leads to a high degree of flexibility in the ordering of tasks).

Tasks refer to person_roles and 'teamaction' items. Teamactions augment operations of creatures or subjects for use in a cooperation context. This way, any item-oriented program can be easily extended for 'cooperation awareness', i.e. for use in a CSCW-type and/or workflow-type cooperation context.

Fig. 3.4 indicates how methods can be augmented for cooperative use. Standard items are shown to the left, subject_roles to the right. The important part is the teamaction context in the middle colomn which determines the choice among different pre-defined alternatives (about synchronism, visibility, and mode) about the cooperative use of the operations.

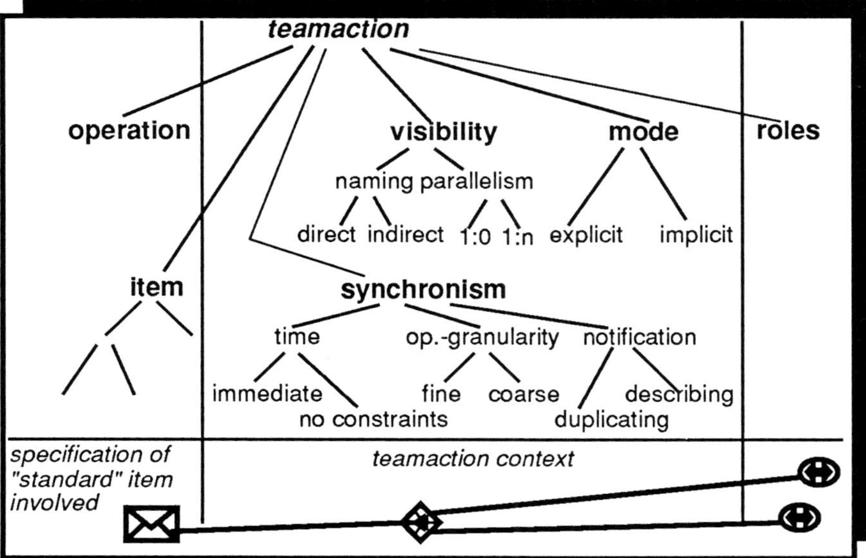

Fig. 3.4: Teamaction context of an item

[Rüd91] explains how these choices cover all kinds of CSCW-interactions available in all CSCW applications known from the literature. The more in-depth discussion in this reference brings evidence to the advantages of the items-oriented cooperation approach over other ones known from the literature. But even from the brief discussion in this section, it should become clear that our approach is neither limited to a specific subset of possible cooperative applications nor concentrates on the CSCW aspects of software engineering alone (such as the [HBP93]), and that it is superiour to class library approaches such as GroupKit [RoG92].

Through the use of subject_roles, a teamaction can refer to an activity without determining whether it is carried out manually or automatic. This way, a workflow can remain unchanged while individual activities are automated in an enterprise.

3.7 Hypertext support

The item categories 'link' and 'navigation' form the basis for hypertext support in the Items system. A serious drawback of existing hypertext systems lies in a lack of typing support. While every hypertext can be interpreted as a graph consisting of 'nodes' and 'links', not all hypertext systems include a sophisticated (e.g., object-oriented) typing concept for such nodes and links; virtually *no* hypertext system supports typing for the hypertext networks (graphs) made up from nodes and links.

Typing support for nodes and links is relatively easy to achieve. In items (where pre-defined types are categories), every sub-category of the subject category can be handled as a 'node type'; every link type must be a sub-category of the relation category and must have the 'link' category as one of its super-categories.

Typing support for hypertext networks, however, is more difficult. The central question is: 'what *is* a network type' (in other words, a 'class' or 'family' of hypertext networks)? In items, we use an approach which was first discussed in the context of a predecessor project [Müh91]. A type of a hypertext network is thereby described as a navigation category, based on a visual graph grammar depiction as indicated in fig. 3.5.

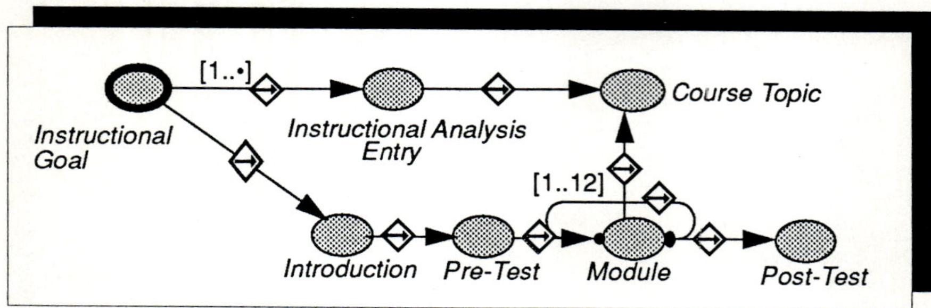

Fig. 3.5. Example hypertext network type

In fig. 3.5, the 'construction' part of a network type (i.e., navigation category) definition is shown. This part describes the rules which determine the graph structure of any hypertext of the respective category. The figure illustrates an example taken from instructional software. The link in the upper left of the figure is marked with an interval [1..°]; this means that at least 1 link of the given type has to originat from the subject 'instructional goal', but there may be as many such links (with the same source node) as desired. In the lower right of the picture, a loop with interval [1..12] is drawn. This shows that in a hypertext of the given category, as many as 12 nodes of type 'Module' may exist in a row, interconnected by the link type indicated in the loop. Apart from the construction rules mentioned, further ones exist of course, as described in [Müh91].

Apart from 'construction' part as just described, a navagation category consists of a 'navigation' part which describs rules and constraints that determine the way in which an individual thread traverses a network of the category described. The experiences with predecessor projects of items have shown that by programming navigation rules in the context of a hypertext category instead of re-programming it for every instance, considerable gains in re-usability and understandability of hypertext-based programs can be made.

4 Summary

We presented an overview of a proposed modeling / programming framework for cooperative media-integrated applications, called Items. The proposal is based on the experience gained with two predecessor frameworks and a sample CMA. It is embedded into a suite of several high-speed networking projects which provide the testbed for our work.

The work described is not completed, but the major conceptual elements have been tested in smaller individual prototype versions of the framework.

References

[Ach91] Achauer, B.:
Distribution in Trellis/DOWL.
Proc. TOOLS 5, Santa Barbara, USA, July 1991, pp. 49 - 59

[ADH93] Altenhofen, M, Dittrich, J., Hammerschmidt, R., et al.:
The BERKOM Multimedia Collaboration Service
Proc. ACM Multimedia '93, 1.-6.8.1993, Anaheim, CA

[Bla92] Blakowski, G.:
High Level Services for Distrib. Multimedia Applications
Based on Application Media and Environment Descriptions.
Proc. ACSC-15, Hobart, Australia, January 1992.
Australian COmputer Science Communications, 14(1), 1992, pp. 93-109

[BHL92] Blakowski, B., Hübel, J., Langrehr, U., Mühlhäuser, M.:
Tool Support for the Synchronization and Presentation of Distributed Multimedia
Butterworth Jl. on Computer Communications, December 1992. pp. 611 - 618

[GZH90] Gerteis, W., Zeidler, Ch., Heuser, L., Mühlhäuser, M.:
DOCASE: A Development Environment & Design Language f. Distrib. O-O
Applications. Proc. TOOLS Pacific '90, Sydney, Australia, Nov. 1990, pp. 298 - 312

[HBP93] Hill, R., Brinck, T., Patterson, J., et al.:
The Rendezvous Language and Architecture
CACM 36 (1), Jan. 1993, pp. 62-67

[Heu90] Heuser, L.:
Processes in Distributed Object-Oriented Applications.
Proc. Tool'90, Karlsruhe, Germany, Nov. 1990, pp. 281 - 290

[Kat93] Katz, S.:
A Superimposition Control Construct for Distributed Systems
ACM ToPLaS 15 (2), April 1993, pp. 337 - 356

[MGH93] Mühlhäuser, M., Gerteis, W., Heuser, L.:
DOCASE - A Methodic Approach to Distributed Object-Oriented Programming
to appear in CACM 36 (10), Sept. 1993

[Müh91] Mühlhäuser, M.:
Hypermedia and Navigation as a Basis for Authoring / Learning Environments
AACE Jl. of Educational Multimedia and Hypermedia, Vol 1, No. 1, 1991, pp. 51 - 64

[MüS92] Mühlhäuser, M., Schaper, J.:
Project Nestor: New Approaches to Cooperative Multimedia Authoring / Learning
in: I. Tomek (Ed.): Computer Assisted Learning, Springer Verlag, Berlin etc. 1992,
pp. 453 - 465

[Pot89] Potts, C.:
Recording the Reasons for Design Decisions.
Proc. IEEE 11th Int. Conf. on SW Engineering, Singapore, May 1989, pp. 418 - 427

[RoG92] Roseman, M., Greenberg, S.:
GroupKit: A Groupware Toolkit for Building Real-Time Conference Applications
Proc. CSCW '92.

[Rüd91] Rüdebusch, T.:
Development and Runtime Support for Collaborative Applications.
in: H.J. Bullinger: Human Aspects in Computing. Elsevier Science Publishers
Amsterdam 1991, pp. 1128 - 1132

[Sch90] Schill, A.:
Mobility Control in Distributed Object-Oriented Applications.
Proc. IEEE Intl. Conf. on Computers and Communications,
Phoenix, Az, March 1989, pp. 395-401.

[ScG90] Schill, A.., Gerteis, W.:
Communication Schedules: An N-Party Communication Abstraction Mechanism for
Distrib. Applications. Proc. 10th ICCC '90 (Nov. 1990, New Delhi, India), pp. 643-651.

The Next Generation of Distributed Multimedia Systems

Ralf Steinmetz
IBM European Networking Center,Vangerowstr.18, 69115 Heidelberg, Germany
Fax: +49-6221-593400, e-mail: steinmet@dhdibmip.bitnet

Abstract

Distributed multimedia systems have been designed and implemented for several computer platforms, operating and window systems. All of them are conceived according to the paradigms of their specific environment. The Unix and the X window system with it's client(Xlib)-server approach is the most frequently used system for multimedia prototypes in the research community.

Interoperability between different systems and vendors are provided by means of common protocols and data (audio and video) coding formats. The next challenge is to conceive system structures for distinct environments which are nicely integrated with the various paradigms. This paper outlines such an approach which is currently under development at IBM ENC, Heidelberg. It provides distributed multimedia services on AIX, it enhances the OS/2 multimedia capabilities for distribution and integrates both as a distributed multimedia system.

Keywords

Multimedia, multimedia communication, distributed systems, distributed multimedia systems

1 Introduction: Environment

At the IBM European Networking Center (ENC) in Heidelberg, Germany, several HeiProjects have been established to develop prototypes that support distributed multimedia applications on RS/6000s under9 AIX as well as on PS/2s under OS/2 / 11/. By "multimedia" we mean that continuous media such as audio and video is always taken into account /33; 33c/. Within this framework we encompass three related areas:

- The *HEIDELBERG CONTINUOUS-MEDIA REALM* (HeiCoRe) is concerned with providing local multimedia services to the applications. The essential services are the resource management and a real-time environment for stream handlers /14/. The resource management negotiates and guarantees the availability of the required resources such as memory, processing, bandwidth and delay. The real-time environment allows to fullfil these requirements by introducing real-time into conventional operating system environments /14/. In the initial phase we designed and implemented this system support for AIX as well as OS/2. Note, as soon as multimedia products such as IBM's Multimedia Presentation Manager/2 (MMPM/2) /17/ became available, we interfaced them replacing earlier prototype code.

- The *HEIDELBERG TRANSPORT SYSTEM* (HeiTS) transfers continuous media data between systems over today's networks such as Token Ring or FDDI in real time. The kind of media and it's properties are specified by the transport service user employing quality of service (QoS) parameters, which are then negotiated between the different HeiTS stacks. HeiTS comprises access to the communication adaptors, ST II as a network layer and HeiTP as a "thin" transport layer. HeiTS runs as a stream handler in the HeiCoRe environment and was the starting point of our integrated multimedia communication system's research and development.
- The *HEIDELBERG MULTIMEDIA APPLICATION TOOLKIT* (HeiMAT) interfaces to HeiCoRe, providing a uniform distribution mechanism on both platforms. It allows for abstractions of multimedia data, implements functions that are commonly needed in multimedia applications like synchronization and mixing of streams, and finally supplies the developer with these application-specific abstractions ready to use. It is aimed to supply AIX as well as OS/2 applications with the same homogeneous interface. This paper outlines the system architecture around HeiMAT which meets the requirements of these two distinct system environments. This is discussed in the framework of the respective evolutionary steps of distributed multimedia systems.

In the research community people sometimes tend to 'reinvent the wheel' as they ignore the evolving products related to their specific topic(s). Concerning audio and video in computing, there exist many 'local' multimedia products, for example, IBM's Multimedia Presentation Manager/2 /17/, Microsoft's Multimedia Extensions /22/ and Apple's Quicktime /4/. In several research driven projects similar capabilities were developed in conjunction with the specific application needs. Distributed multimedia systems should make use of these products by interfacing the available components.

Several experimental systems provide HeiMAT like functions. Among them are ACME /2/ VOX /1/, and Sventek's system /34/. Unlike HeiMAT, they are based solely on one environment which differentiates our system somewhat. One goal of the HeiProjects was to show this is not an insurmountable problem, rather a further abstraction from the system details.

Section 2 reviews the initial steps in distributed multimedia systems with a "hybrid" system structure, and Section 3 provides an overview of "unified" systems. In the next section the design demands as well as the available environments on two distinct platforms are outlined.

2 "Hybrid" System Structures

Early prototypes of distributed and local multimedia systems, such as the Integrated Media Architecture Laboratory (IMAL), conceived at Bell Communications Research in Red Bank /21/; or the Muse and Pygmalion system of MIT's Project Athena /16; 5; 26/, were based on a "hybrid" system structure /13/. In this framework, continuous media is mainly processed by devices located outside of the workstations. Most of the real-time processing is performed by dedicated processors and not by the main CPU(s). Traditionally, instead of sending video data to a workstation via a LAN for presentation in a window on the display, video data is sent over dedicated channels to a separate video monitor as shown in Figure 1. These devices are, however, attached to the workstation and controlled by the workstation's software.

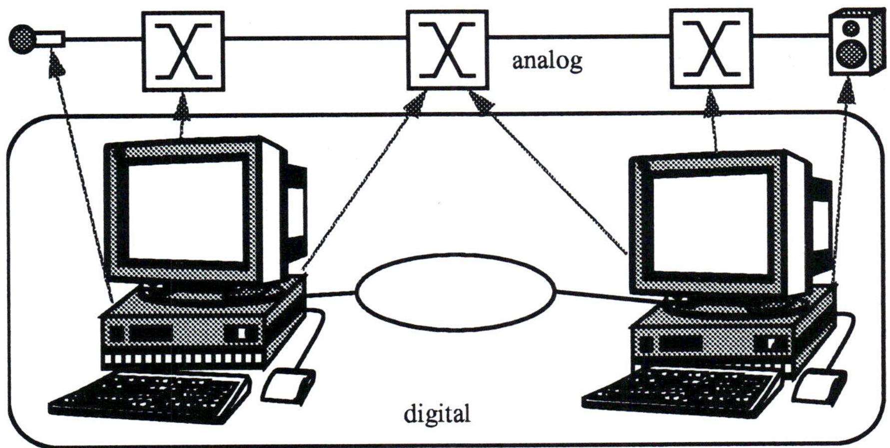

Figure 1: Hybrid System

The DiME (Distributed Multimedia Environment) project, carried out at the ENC in Heidelberg, was based on such a hybrid system structure. Continuous media is routed over dedicated channels using off-the-shelf hardware technology. Continuous and discrete media were integrated by connecting the audio and video equipment (e.g., CD players, VCRs) to a computer via an RS-232C interface. Devices could have been incorporated into the system as additional boards, for instance, the audio/video data was processed in the workstation using IBM's AVC and M-Motion adapters with respective system software /24; 23/. Further experiments included the ActionMedia 750 and ActionMedia II (DVI) technology /8/ for grabbing of images out of a video stream. DiME dealt with distributed, transparent access to multimedia resources like cameras and stored video sequences /27; 28; 29/. It aimed to provide an “easy, but rich” communication service as part of an application programming interface, manipulating data streams by controlling their sources and sinks in a heterogeneous computing environment. Synchronization has been a key issue in multimedia systems, it was also addressed in DiME by control of the devices located at the sources and sinks /31/.

Hybrid system structures require cost overheads for the additional devices not being part of the workstations, e.g., the required interconnections do not make use of available computer networks. The upgrade of a small system with about 10 involved workstations to a larger set-up with, e.g., more than 50 computers requires a considerable redesign of the hardware configuration, ‘right-sizing’ is difficult. In this hybrid approach the computer handles continuous media devices rather than the continuous media data. The audio and video data does not enter the computer after being generated; rather it passes through separate devices and it’s own communication lines. Furthermore, continuous media data can not be manipulated with a fine granularity, operations like ‘start’ and ‘stop’ are supported.

This leads to some dedicated problems, for example, in synchronization. It is very difficult to achieve tight synchronization between discrete and continuous media. Discrete media and continuous media data are transmitted over different networks and processing nodes having different end-to-end delay characteristics. End-to-end delay over continuous media paths is typically shorter than for discrete media. By experiment, it is difficult and expensive (in terms of buffer capacity) to delay continuous media data delivered from devices like cameras or microphones. If discrete media is faster than continuous media, buffering and time stamping can be used to slow down the data stream, however these situations very rarely occur /32/.

3 “Unified” System Structures

The control of continuous media can be more immediate if all data passes through the computer system itself. This is only possible with digital data encoding. One of the first systems featuring digital audio in a computer environment was the Etherphone system developed at XEROX PARC /35/ in which an Ethernet is used for data communication and telephony. A similar early approach was used in a project by AT&T in Naperville /19; 20/ where a fast packet-switching network was directly attached to workstations. Enhancements to the UNIX operating system introduced the notion of "connectors" and "active devices" for handling continuous media.

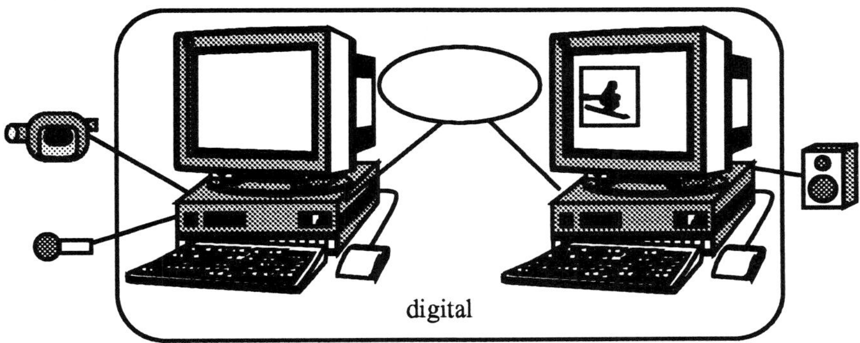

Figure 2: Unified System

Our follow-on project in it's first phase, the Heidelberg High-Speed Transport System (HeiTS), is based on this unified digital system structure /9/. Scheduling of continuous media data can either be done exclusively in software and/or by dedicated hardware, such as the ActionMedia II board (DVI). Both solutions require real-time techniques in a time-sharing environment (/10; 25/ similar to /3/).

Most of today's systems being conceived and implemented follow this approach. The design of the distributed systems follows the paradigms available in the respective environment. The communication between such systems is made possible by using the same protocols for continuous media, for example, ST II /12/ with HeiTP /7/, or a multimedia capable XTP /30/. The challenges of the next generation is to design and implement system structures which are appropriate for different computer architectures.

4 "Cross-Platform" System Structures

For the services provided by such an approach we foresee the following demands /15/:

- At the highest level it should be very *easy to develop applications*. The distributed system layer requires only the essential knowledge from the application in order to supply the demanded services. Then it takes care of all the details involved with establishment of data streams using devices in the distributed system.
- Coding technology is still evolving today, and it appears that committee stan-

dards compete with de-facto standards, where various implementations provide distinct algorithms for the same coding applications /33b/. The ISO JPEG standard defines compression and coding of single images like many available de-facto standards. The ISO MPEG video specification defines compression and to some extent competes with the CCITT H.261 and the DVI de-facto compression standard. MPEG-2 is still to be defined for video compression with higher quality. MPEG audio as well as the CCITT G.721 and 722 proposals are aimed at audio compression. Applications need to be developed without constraining to certain coding techniques by making use of the *presentation transparency* of the distributed system layer.

- Application must not see any difference in interfacing local or remote devices. By this *distribution transparency* the applications do not need to know explicitly the location of devices. Certainly by some applications it is required to be aware of the location and, e.g., to handle properly security aspects. Therefore, for the application it should be possible to make use of this knowledge but, only if it is required.

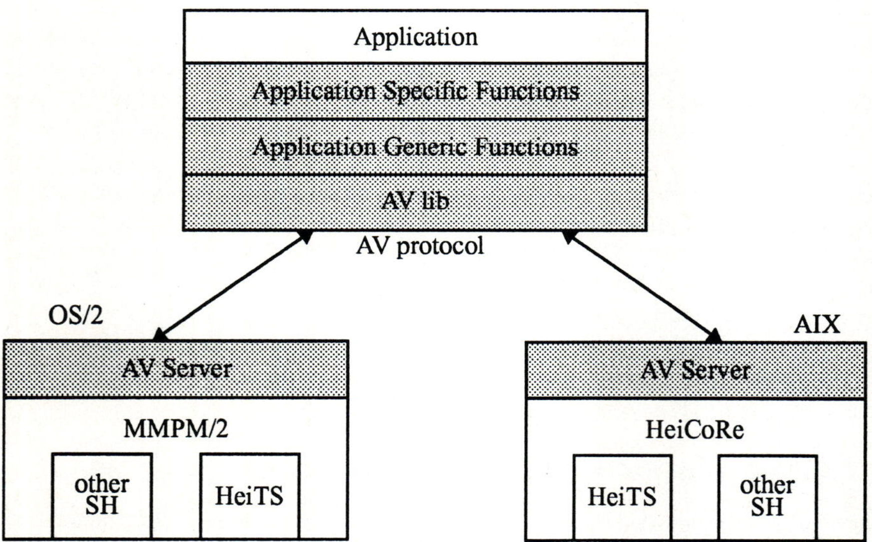

Figure 3: Cross-Platform Architecture

The *independence from multimedia devices* means to hide the characteristics of physical devices, allowing for the development of portable applications. For the remote control of a camera in order to change the position or to adjust the focus, most of the available camera control units require different interfaces. Some of them operate on a type of 'start and stop' semantics: the application is able to initiate or stop the movement. At other interfaces it is possible to specify the relative movement in term of, e.g., 'move north by 10 degrees'. Application programming should be independent of such implementation details. As a major interface metaphor, the application program interface should includes the notion of sources, sinks and streams.

This set of demands together with the distinct environments of the two different platforms impose hard design requirements on the system structure. The envisaged distributed system layer (HeiMAT) has to be a seamless integrator of the available paradigms on both platforms. The system structure is shown in the illustration above.

The OS/2 platform provides the MMPM/2 as the local multimedia extension to the operating system. MMPM/2 already allows the definition of sources and sinks of streams. HeiCoRe is used to add the resource management, it provides the reservation and scheduling of reserved resources in a distributed system taking into account the characteristics of the networks /36/. MMPM/2 closely interacts with the IBM's Presentation Manager which was designed for fast response times with a large set of functions in a local environment.

For the input and output of discrete media in a distributed UNIX environment, the X window system is the most widely used system. The layered approach of X is encompassing a client server approach. We envisage the multimedia support in a distributed environment to be architected in a similar manner to X. A continuous media server - which we call the AV server - communicates with the window system for presentation on the common display. The AV server encapsulates the functionality of HeiCoRe providing access to all types of stream-oriented multimedia devices/filters through a consistent interface. Native HeiCoRe applications coexist with the AV server and can interface to HeiCoRe. Similar to X, the communication between server and client is supported by an AV protocol which itself is hidden by an AVlib. A typical function set provided by the AVlib will include operations for creation, modification, connection, control, and destruction of the logical multimedia devices. These devices operate in a dedicated real-time environment. HeiMAT interfaces the AV server through the AVlib which can be seen as encapsulated into HeiMAT. Using this AVlib interface, HeiMAT will provide a higher-level API allowing for easy development of distributed multimedia applications. A prototype of the AV server and AVlib was developed in an object oriented C++ framework. This basic level of HeiMAT is, therefore, analogous to the X toolkit level.

However, HeiMAT will also support the development of multimedia interfaces through special widget sets similar to OSF/Motif. OS/2 already incorporates these through MMPM/2 /18/. These widgets provide the user of applications the same 'look and feel' for different multimedia applications. For this purpose in AIX, HeiMAT uses the X toolkit stack in conjunction with the AV server to provide it's services.

The Media Control Interface is the native OS/2 MMPM/2 component to be interfaced by applications. For the distribution of this interface an X-like server is being built around this native OS/2 Interface. It is known as the 'AV Server' which distributes the remote calls to the local multimedia devices via the Media Control Interface. Handles of the Presentation Manager's functions, which are used in the MMPM/2, can not be passed transparently as this window system has no client/server architecture such as X. Therefore the windowing application in OS/2 will always run at the client's station. In the first release of the distributed OS/2 system, HeiCam (Heidelberg Remote Camera Control) uses this transparent distributed access to remote multimedia devices.

As an alternative to our solution the distribution can be hidden under the Media Control Interface within the MMPM/2. There, at least two approaches can be followed:

- Each Media Driver establishes it's own communication with the remote entity(ies). As a consequence, there exist local as well as distributed Media Drivers. In our experiments it turned out that the commonalities of the various distributed Media Drivers are not taken into account. It must also be mentioned that no general scheme to name and to address the respective remote services exists.
- All kind of distribution is performed via the file system. In terms of OS/2 (unlike UNIX) all devices are not seen as being of similar input-output nature. The stream handlers are the sources and sinks of continuous data and, the file system is just one of these stream handlers. This approach is a suitable alternative for homogenous environments which focus on storage and retrieval applications. In such an approach the control of a remote cameras is handled similar to the access to files. At the programming interface we experienced that it is easier to operate on streams, sinks and sources than only on files. Therefore we did not follow this approach.

Due to the mentioned reasons we decide to build a server around the local multimedia functions and did not add distribution capabilities to individual entities within this multimedia extension.

In our Heidelberg multimedia system, the HeiRAT component /36/ is in charge of the resource management. HeiRAT accepts quality of service (QoS) requests from the AVlib (as part of HeiMAT). HeiRAT can be seen as part of the AVserver which serves for the QoS demands as interface to the whole distributed system. It makes use of the ST II flow specification to negotiate them among the whole set of involved system components /7b/. It provides a QoS calculation by optimizing one QoS parameter dependent on the resource characteristics. Subsequently resources are reserved according to the QoS guarantees. At the actual data transfer phase resources are scheduled (in the real-time environment) to provide these guarantees.

As a part of the HeiProjects we architected this system structure and defined HeiMAT to be the encapsulation of the client multimedia library. However, HeiMAT goes beyond the existing multimedia services of MMPM/2 and the related AVlib interfaces in providing abstractions such as a video conferencing module that serves as a building block for multimedia applications.

5 Conclusion

Distributed multimedia system structures evolved from *hybrid* to *unified* approaches. In several European projects around ESPRIT, RACE and DELTA as well as in national initiatives like BERKOM /37/, systems are implemented which interconnect UNIX and UNIX-like environments of different vendors. The next generation will comprise *cross-platform* solutions which additionally cover different system environments like AIX and OS/2.

This paper discusses an approach of such a cross-platform solution. Implementation of different basic components as well as the design of upper layer toolkit like modules is in progress. A first system, together with a conferencing application was shown at COMDEX, Las Vegas, November 1992 and at CeBIT, March 1993. The current version (demonstrated at CeBIT'93) includes the main ideas as outlined in this paper.

As a matter of fact we were forced to provide the interoperability of the different platforms, therefore, in order to avoid a duplication of work we developed this concept of portability and interoperability between various platforms. We experienced that the concept of the AVlib and AVserver is excellent to meet the requirements of ease of development, distribution transparency, presentation transparency and independence from multimedia devices. We see no reason why our system can not be ported to non-IBM platforms.

We are still in the phase of redesign of the interface to the application including the Application Specific and Generic Functions. We have two different environments and implementations which we are still not satisfied with. Each approach tends to either be very effective and closely related to one specific operating system environment or it tends to be too generic for being efficient to implement a whole set of different applications on various machines. It is still an open issue how such an excellent interface in terms of, e.g., an object oriented class hierarchy should look like in order to support the set of interactive as well as retrieval like multimedia applications.

I would like to thank all the application and applications support teams which are in charge of the distributed system in the HeiProjects. Thomas Käppner provided his in-depth X and UNIX experience in designing a toolkit approach for HeiMAT. Jürgen Falter and Peter Sander contributed with their MMPM/2 experience. Thomas Meyer reminded us of all possible obstacles and helped with his exceptional multimedia synchronization and abstractions experience. Ralf Guido Herrtwich intensively pushed all the initial steps and discussed in detail many issues of system structure. Dietmar Hehmann made extensive use of his profound OS/2 as well as AIX background in order to get an aligned solution for both systems. Ian Marsh provided substantial contributions to the whole paper in it's final version.

6 References

/1/ B. Arons, C. Binding, K. Lantz, C. Schmandt. The VOX Audio Server. 2nd IEEE COMSOC International Multimedia Communications Workshop, Montebello, Quebec, Canada, Apr. 1989.

/2/ David Anderson, Pamela Chan; Toolkit Support for Multiuser Audio/Video Applications; 2nd International Workshop on Network and Operating System Support for Digital Audio and Video, Heidelberg, November 18-19, 1991.

/3/ David P. Anderson; Meta-Scheduling for Distributed Continuous Media; Computer Science Division (EECS) Report No. UCB/CSD 90/599, U. C. Berkeley, Berkeley CA, October 1990.

/4/ Apple; QuickTime Developer's Kit Version 1.0; Apple Document Number 030-1899.

/5/ George Champine, Daniel Geer, William Ruh; Project Athena as a Distributed Computer System; IEEE Computer, vol.23 no.9, September 1990, pp.40-51.

/6/ Andreas Cramer, Manny Farber, Brain McKellar Ralf Steinmetz; Experiences with the Heidelberg Multimedia Communication System: Multicast, Rate Enforcement and Performance; IFIP European High Performance Networking Workshop (ehpn'92), Liege, Belgium, December 1992.

/7/ Luca Delgrossi, Christian Halsstrick, Ralf Guido Herrtwich, Heiner Stuettgen; HeiTP - A Transport Protocol for ST-II; IBM ENC Technical Report, 1992.

/7b/ Luca Delgrossi, Ralf Guido Herrtwich, Frank Oliver Hoffmann: An Implementation of ST-II for the Heidelberg Transport System, IBM Technical Report 43.9303, IBM European Networking Center, Heidelberg, 1993.

/8/ Kevin Harney, Mike Keith, Gary Lavelle, Lawrence D. Ryan, Daniel J. Stark; The i750 Video processor: A Total Multimedia Solution; Communications of the ACM, vol.34, no.4, April 1991, pp.64-78.

/9/ Dietmar Hehmann, Ralf Guido Herrtwich, Werner Schulz, Thomas Schuett, Ralf Steinmetz; HeiTS - Architecture and Implementation of the Heidelberg High-Speed Transport System; 2nd International Workshop on Network and Operating System Support for Digital Audio and Video, Heidelberg, November 18-19, 1991.

/10/ Ralf Guido Herrtwich; The Role of Performance, Scheduling, and Resource Reservation in Multimedia Systems; Proc. Operating Systems in the Nineties and Beyond, Lecture Notes of Computer Science, Springer, 1991.

/11/ Ralf Guido Herrtwich; The HeiProjects: Support for Distributed Multimedia Applications; IBM Technical Report, no.43.9206, March 1992.

/12/ Ralf Guido Herrtwich; The Evolution of ST II; Position Paper for the Dagstuhl Seminar, Novembner 1992.

/13/ Lutz Henkel, Heinrich J. Stuettgen; Transportdienste in Breitbandnetzen; GI Conference, Communication in Distributed Systems, Mannheim, Germany, E. Effelsberg, H.W. Meuer, G. Mueller (Ed), Springer Verlag, pp.96-111, February, 1991.

/14/ Ralf Guido Herrtwich, Lars Wolf; A System Software Structure for Distributed Multimedia Systems; 5th Acontinuous media SIGOPS European Workshop, Le Mont Saint-Michel, France, September 1992.

/15/ Dietmar Hehmann, Thomas Kaeppner, Ralf Steinmetz; An Introduction to HeiMAT: The Heidelberg Multimedia Application Toolkit 3rd International Workshop on Network and Operating System Support for Digital Audio and Video, San Diego, CA, Nov. , 1992.

/16/ Matthew E. Hodges, Russel M. Susnett, Mark S. Ackerman; A Construction Set for Multimedia Applications; IEEE Software Magazine, January 1989, pp. 37-43.

/17/ IBM; Multimedia Presentation Manager/2: Programming Reference; IBM Document From Number 41G2920, 1992.

/18/ Thomas Käppner; Personal Communication; August 1992.

/19/ Wu-Hon F. Leung, Gottfried W. R. Luderer; The Network Operating System Concept for Future Services; AT & T Technical Journal, vol.68, no.2, April 1989, pp. 23-35.

/20/ W.H. Leung, T.J. Baumgartner, Y.H. Hwang, M.J. Morgan, S. C. Tu. A Software Architecture for Workstation Supporting Multimedia Conferencing in Packet Switching Networks. IEEE Journal on Selected Areas in Communication, vol.8, no.3, April 1990, pp. 380-390.

/21/ L.F.Ludwig, D.F.Dunn; Laboratory for Emulation and Study of Integrated and Coordinated Media Communication; Frontiers in Computer Technology, Proc. of the ACM SIGCOMM '87 Workshop, August 11-13,1987.

/22/ Microsoft Corporation; Microsoft Windows Multimedia Programmer's Reference; Microsoft Press, 1991.

/23/ M-Motion Video Adapter/A, User's Guide, Product Description; IBM 1990.

/24/ Daniel J. Moore; Multimedia Presentation Development using the Audio Visual Connection; IBM Systems Journal, Vol.29, No.4, 1990, pp.494-508.

/25/ Andreas Mauthe, Werner Schulz, Ralf Steinmetz; Inside the Heidelberg Multimedia Operating System Support: Real-Time Processing of Continuous Media in OS/2; IBM ENC Technical Report, October 1992.

/26/ W.E. Mackay, W. Treese, D. Applebaum, B. Gardner, B. Michon, E. Schlusselberg, M. Ackermann, D. Davis Pygmalion: An Experiment in Multimedia Communication Proceedings of SIGGRAPH 89, Boston, July 1989.

/27/ Johannes Rueckert, Hermann Schmutz, Bernd Schoener, Ralf Steinmetz; A Distributed Multimedia Environment for Advanced CSCW Applications; IEEE Multimedia '90, Bordeaux, November 15-17, 1990.

/28/ Ralf Steinmetz, Reinhard Heite, Johannes Rueckert, Bernd Schoener; Compound Multimedia Objects - Integration into Network and Operating Systems; International Workshop on Network and Operating System Support for Digital Audio and Video, International Computer Science Institute, Berkeley, November 8-9, 1990.

/29/ Bernd Schoener, Johannes Rueckert, Ralf Steinmetz; Media Related Requirements for Communication Services; 6th IEEE International Workshop on Telematics, Corea, September 1991.

/30/ Jochen Sandvoss, Thomas Schuett, Markus Steffen, Ralf Steinmetz; XTP und Multimedia?; GI Conference, Communication in Distributed Systems, Muenchen 1993.

/31/ Ralf Steinmetz; Synchronization Properties in Multimedia Systems; IEEE Journal on Selected Areas in Communication, vol. 8, no. 3, April 1990, pp. 401-412.

/32/ Ralf Steinmetz, Multimedia Synchronization Techniques: Experiences Based on Different System Structures; IEEE Multimedia Workshop '92, Monterey, CA, USA, April'92.

/33/ Ralf Steinmetz, Ralf Guido Herrtwich; Integrierte verteilte Multimedia-Systeme; Informatik Spektrum, Springer Verlag, vol.14, no.5, October 1991, pp.280-282.

/33b/ Ralf Steinnmetz; Compression Techniques in Multimedia Systems; IBM ENC Technical Report no.43.9305, 1993; and accepted for publication in acm/Springer Multimedia Systems Journal, 1994.

/33c/ Ralf Steinmetz; Multimedia-Technology: Introduction and Fundamentals (book, in German); Springer-Verlag, October 1993.

/34/ J.S.Sventek; An Architecture for Supporting Multimedia Integration; IEEE Computer Society Office Automatition Symposium, April 1987, pp.46-56.

/35/ Daniel C. Swinehart; Telephone Management in the Etherphone System; IEEE Globecom'87, 1987, pp. 30.3.1-30.3.5.

/36/ Carsten Vogt, Ralf Guido Herrtwich, Ramesh Nagarajan; HeiRAT: The Heidelberg Resource Administration Technique, Design Philosophy and Goals; IBM ENC Technical Report no.43.9101, 1991.

/37/ BERKOM Breitband Kommunuikation im Glasfasernetz; H.Ricke, J.Kanzow (Hsrg.), R. v. Decker's Verlag, 1991.

Third Section

Finegrained Synchronisation in Dynamic Documents

Wolfgang Herzner
Dept. for Information Technology
Austrian Research Centre Seiberdorf
A-2444 Seiberdorf

Abstract: Dynamic documents not only contain 'dynamic' contents like videos, audios, or animation, but more generally, changes over time during their presentation as well as temporal dependencies among components play a crucial role for them. Lectures and exams in computer-based education, entertainment (games), and even simulation are considered as target application areas. Authors of those documents (or applications, respectively) must be able to describe such temporal relationships. Therefore, an event-based model is presented, which not only allows one to specify synchronisational aspects in a flexible way, but also supports the development of distributed applications, where adjustments for delays caused by hardware and/or software can be considered automatically. In addition, various kinds of user interaction with a document's presentation are also supported. A prototype, which is based on DECpresent (DEC 1990), is currently under implementation at Seibersdorf.

Keywords: Multimedia, Document processing, Synchronisation

1 Introduction

With the availability of cheap and fast hardware for recording and playing video and acoustic information with the computer, accompanied by appropriate software, there is actually some evidence that multimedia components are going to become integral part of computing environments, as has happened with spreadsheets or electronic publishing in the past few years. Although the 'accompanying' basic software usually merely deals with recording, editing, and presenting of a single medium – audio or video, it is sufficient for all kinds of applications where the isolated presentation of these media is sufficient. This the more as graphical user interfaces ('GUI') usually permit the presentation of videos together with other information on the same screen. In addition, *hyper-links* (Gloor and Streitz 1990, DEC 1991, Hahn et al. 1992) can serve to associate dynamic media with conventional ones. Combining these ingredients already provide a basic environment for presenting multimedia information.

It is, however, sometimes necessary to specify more precisely how different pieces of information are related, both in space – layout – and time – synchronisation. For example, in an advertising presentation of a new product, the movie showing the product shall not appear just anywhere on the screen, but in a certain frame within a window containing other, i.e. static, information. And some sound shall be played (e.g. a 'splash') whenever a certain condition becomes true (e.g. an animated character hits a water surface).

Since this is reminiscent of the layout process of conventional documents, such applications shall be referred to as *dynamic documents* in this paper. At least the following application areas are considered:

— computer-based training and education,
— product presentation,
— entertainment,
— simulation.

Remark: due to the high interactivity of a user with the presentation of some information, as well as the inclusion of animation, the border between 'document' and 'application' actually has become fuzzy. But since this paper concentrates on the presentation of permanently stored information, emphasis is laid on the 'document' aspect (as reflected in the title).

An aspect currently strongly increasing in importance, is that of distributed computing environments. In our context, this primarily means that information will be distributed over a network; but it also implies that applications themselves may be distributed. Besides multi-player games, consider a training program, where the teacher gets informed automatically about the progress of their students (located at different nodes).

So, the following aspects of dynamic documents can be identified:

a) Conventional layout.
b) Complex temporal constraints, e.g.:
   — "*show object A when one of the events* $E_1, .., E_m$ *occurs, but none of the conditions* $C_1, .., C_n$ *is true*".
c) User-interaction, e.g.:
   — control playing speed of several objects with a 'slider', which shall be part of the document;
   — the user shall answer a question within a certain time frame (by 'clicking' a button).
d) Hardware and software related delays, e.g.:
   — positioning of CD-players;
   — transmission of remotely stored content.
e) Distributed presentation, e.g.:
   — "*display some information at screen A, when the user at B performed a certain action*".
f) Spatial-temporal relationships, e.g.:
   — "*do not overlap simultaneously shown videos*";
   — "*move object A along a path P according to progression of object B's presentation*".

In the last few years, a number of socalled *multimedia authoring systems* became available (e.g. AimTech 1992, Asymetrix 1991, Authorware 1992, MacroMind 1990), which address the synchronisation aspects listed above with different approaches and to different extents. They usually support (not too complex) synchronisation and animation in an often surprisingly easy way. However, they also tend to share some limitations: they are mostly dedicated for single-user applications, often with one window/screen at a time; delays are not treated very carefully, and they are sometimes not very flexible in modelling user interactions.

To overcome these weak points, an approach shall be presented, which covers or at least addresses these topics. It is based on results of earlier investigations (Kummer and Kuhn 1991, Herzner and Kummer 1992). First, Sect. 2 provides a short overview about methods of existing authoring tools. Then, the synchronisation model itself is discussed in Sect. 3, while Sect. 4 deals with some aspects of the ongoing implementation, including several examples to illustrate the usage of the proposed model. And finally, in Sect. 5, conclusions are summarized.

2 Synchronisation Metaphors

For the specification of temporal dependencies, at least three major approaches or 'metaphors' can be identified in existing authoring tools:

a) Scripts: A textual representation is used to describe temporal constraints, often in a 'natural-language like' formal grammar. Scripts are usually associated with individual objects, rather than one script for the whole document. For example, in the script language OpenScript of the Multimedia ToolBook (Asymetrix 1991), a statement like

```
to handle buttonUp
  go to next page
end buttonUp
```

will advance the presentation to the next page when the user releases the mouse button.

Similar to programming languages, scripts can be very powerful, but are sometimes judged as not user-friendly or being reserved to the professional.

b) Time Lines or Story Boards: Along a time axis, which is often subdivided into smaller units, and which may have different durations, several tracks are provided where specific objects or actions can be entered, as shown in Fig. 2.1a. While appearing to be relatively easy to be used, they tend to show limitations in flexibility, although in combination with scripts, this can be improved. For example, the MacroMind Director (MacroMind 1990) uses this metaphor for the general layout of a presentation, while providing the additional script language Lingo for details.

c) Flow Charts: Presenting objects as icons and synchronisation or data flow as edges between these objects, flow charts not only seem to reflect principles of modern GUIs best, but may also be less limited in flexibility than story boards. On the other hand, complex situations tend to overload such representations, and several aspects which cannot be presented well graphically (e.g. names or iteration counters), are either treated as annotations or hidden in scripts. Authorware Professional (Authorware 1992) and IconAuthor (AimTech 1992), from which Fig. 2.1b is taken, are examples for these approaches.

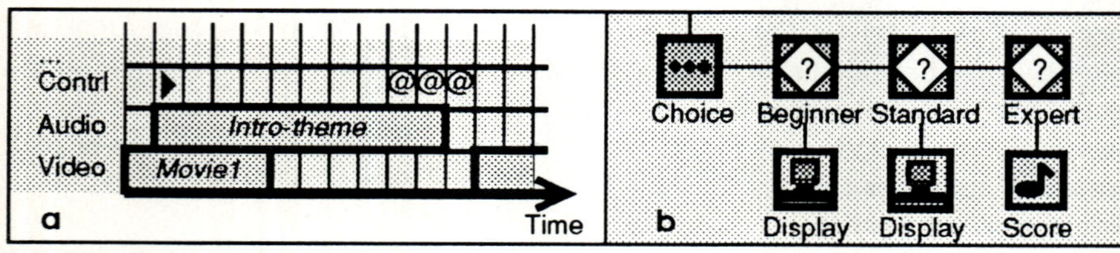

Fig. 2.1. Examples for synchronisation metaphors

3 The Synchronisation Model

This section discusses the generic aspects of the introduced model. For explaining why the described approach has been taken, the requirements taken into consideration are briefly summarized:

— it should be easy to describe simple cases, but
— complex constraints should be efficiently specifiable,
— suitable for various document architectures,
— suitable for various presentation metaphors,
— support of distributed applications,
— support of various types of user interaction.

Now, the generic model departs into following main concepts:

- Document structure (Sect. 3.1)
- Presentation units (Sect. 3.2)
- Directives (Sect. 3.3)
- Input (Sect. 3.4)

Please note that textual examples contained in this section, which are printed in helvetica, do not constitute a real syntax, since this whole section mainly concentrates on conceptual aspects. A number of realisations can be envisioned; one is outlined in the Sect. 4.2.

3.1 Document Structure

To make possible both the applicability of the presented model to a variety of document architectures and the specification of simple synchronisation types like 'parallel' and 'sequential' easy, the following structuring of a document's content is assumed:

- A *document* consists of a set of identifiable *content objects* or *components*, which may include those serving for *input*. The document itself is regarded as the uppermost content element.

- Each content object itself is either *basic* or may consist of a set of subordinate components, which applies recursively.
- Within each set, each component can be presented independently from each other; but any component of a content object can only be presented while the content object itself is presented.
- For each (subset of) such a set, *presentation units* (Sect. 3.2) can be defined, which describe the behaviour of the selected content objects at presentation time.
- Each such set may be ordered sequentially.
- For identifying parts of basic content objects (e.g. frames of videos, words of paragraphs), these objects constitute their individual 'finite coordinate spaces', as described in HyTime (ISO/IEC 1992). If sets of content objects are ordered, then this applies to them as well, by implication.

This leads to a hierarchical multi-level document architecture as indicated in Fig. 3.1.

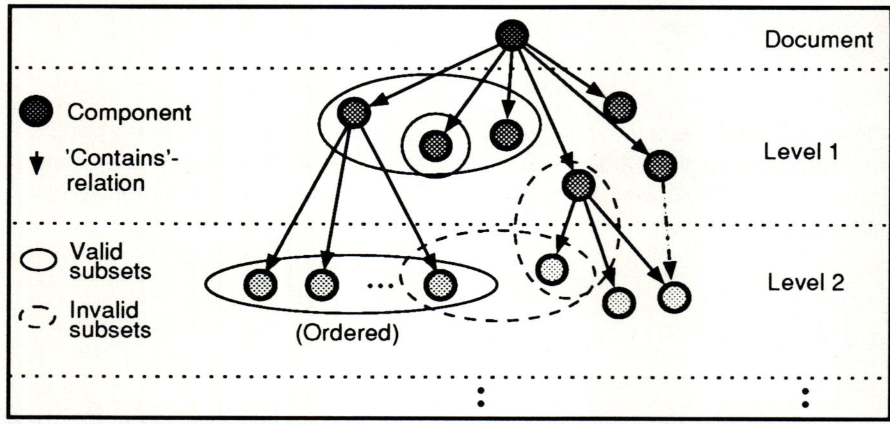

Fig. 3.1. Generic document content structure

<u>Examples</u>:

'Classical document', consisting of chapters, sections, paragraphs, ...
Completely ordered; chapters, sections, etc. map to different levels.

Set of slides. Ordered or unordered, where each slide may have several components, which are representable independently from each other. Level 1 for slides, lower level for nested components.

Set of hyper-link nodes. Unordered; one level, but lower levels within nodes possible.

Remark: Content objects of a set may be distributed over a network, they may be shared within a document (as indicated by the dashed arrow) as well as by several documents.

3.2 Presentation Units

Presentation units (or 'p-units', for short) serve for the description of specific behaviour of content objects at presentation time. For having some content object participating in a presentation, a p-unit must exist which controls that content object. If a component is not controlled by any p-unit, then it will not be presented. This may appear to make things more complicated than necessary, but since nested components are always implicitely included, the creation of one p-unit for the document itself usually will result in the presentation of the whole document.

A content object may be controlled by more than one p-unit. Since an arbitrary number of p-units may be active at the same time, this implies that several instances of a content object may be presented simultaneously. But the primary purpose for that concept is to allow one content object to be presented in different contexts. For example, a slide could be used in several lectures of a course (e.g. Petricek and Zeiler 1991), or a logo could be displayed both at begin and end of a presentation.

The basic characteristics of a p-unit are:

- It has always a certain *sync-type*, given by its *class* (Sect. 3.2.1), which defines the default behaviour.
- It can have a *name* for identification.
- Its *scope* (Sect. 3.2.2) is always a content object or a non-empty subset of its components.
- A *state model* (Sect. 3.2.3) controls its life cycle.
- *Attributes* (Sect. 3.2.4) control additional aspects like 'maximum number of iterations'.
- *Variables* (Sect. 3.2.5) definable by the author provide further control.
- It communicates with other p-units by emitting signals and receiving messages or applying commands, respectively. This is specified by means of *directives*.

To reduce the amount of the author's work, this list also applies to basic content objects. These could therefore be regarded as having p-units of corresponding class automatically associated. For example, to control a video individually, no p-unit needs to be defined for it explicitely, because it can be addressed directly in directives.

This idea can be generalized to all content objects, including the whole document. Then, when creating a non-basic content object, its default sync-type would be selected, which would imply its automatic presentation. Therefore, if such a default is defined for the document itself, it can be presented without specifying any p-unit explicitely. See also Sect. 3.5 for a summary of default rules.

Since the scope of a p-unit can be interpreted as its components, we will – in context with synchronisation – treat p-units and content-objects uniformly. The general term *object* shall denote both for the rest of this paper.

3.2.1 P-unit Classes / Sync-Types

P-unit classes are templates for synchronisation types, from which p-units (and, possibly, also content objects) are instantiated. They can be predefined or specified by the author. Several classes are considered to be of general usage and should therefore be predefined:

parallel: all components are presented in parallel.
loop: like parallel, but restarts automatically.
sequence: like loop, but only one component is presented per iteration. The order is either predefined or given together with the p-unit.

Other classes could be added or derived from existing ones.

3.2.2 Scope

A p-unit is always defined for a content-object or some subset of its components. These are called the scope of the p-unit. In Fig. 3.1, solid ellipses show some examples of valid scopes, while dashed ellipses are examples for invalid ones (contain members of more than one set). A content object which is in the scope of a p-unit is controlled by this p-unit. A scope can be ordered, which is necessary for certain sync-types like sequence.

If a content object, which lies within the scope of some p-unit A, contains components, for which another p-unit B is defined, then B is regarded subordinate to A. In Fig. 3.1, the solid ellipse at level 2 represents a scope of a p-unit, which is subordinate to that of the larger solid ellipse at level 1. Subordinate p-units describe the behaviour of the components within their scope under the scope of their higher p-unit(s).

3.2.3 State Model

During presentation, each object passes through a sequence of *states*. State transitions occur either due to the reaction on received messages (see Sect. 3.3) or due to internal events. In each state, the object performs certain actions, and reacts only on specific messages. At certain state transitions, signals are emitted to indicate the completion of corresponding actions.

Figure 3.2 represents the state diagram, where shaded states allow for adjustment of hard/software caused delays. Message-arrows indicate the latest states along the cascade where the corresponding messages are accepted. This means that, for example, the message start is ignored when received in a state later than is_prepared. However, a start received in state is_idle, will cause an implicit preparation. The message/signal pairs prepare/prepared, start/started, and stop/terminated correspond to the *cues* as introduced in (Herzner W., Kummer, M., 1992). A parallel-object is prepared/started/terminated, when all its components are **prepared/started/terminated**, respectively. For the other sync-types, analogous rules are defined.

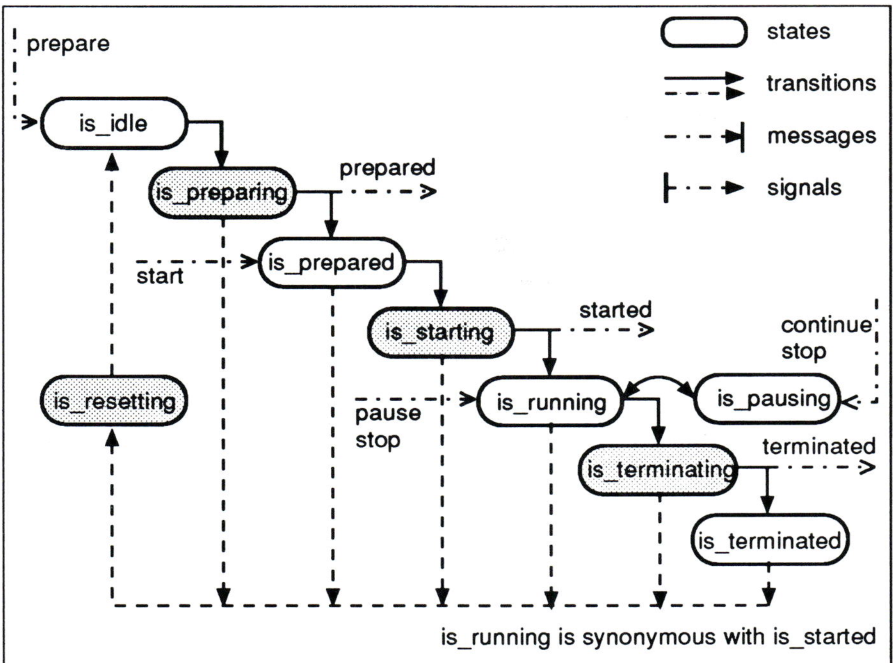

Fig. 3.2. Life cycle state diagram

Once an object has arrived at state **is_terminated**, it cannot be presented anymore, as long as it is not reset, either implicitely by default or a higher iterating object, or explicitely by receiving a **reset** message.

Besides those shown in Fig. 3.2, objects may accept further messages and emit additional signals. For example, iterating objects (e.g. of sync-type **loop** or **sequence**) will stop the current iteration and start the next or the previous one, when receiving **next** or **previous**, respectively. And input objects (Sect. 3.4) may emit the signal **triggered** for indicating a corresponding user action.

3.2.4 Attributes

Each object possesses a number of attributes according to its class or sync-type, which describe or control special characteristics. Depending on their semantics, the author may initialize them, or even specify a rule which controls their values at presentation time. See Sect. 4.2a for a specific example. And their values may be inquired by the *conditions* of *directives* (Sect. 3.3.1). Some examples for attributes are:

pacing: initial value for a pacing factor for all affected dynamic components, applied to normal playing speed.
duration: limits presentation time (per life cycle of one iteration).
max_iteration: limits repetitions of iterating objects.
curr_index: indicates the index of the component currently presented in 'single-component-at-a-time' iterations.
autoreset: indicates whether the object shall be reset automatically after termination.
round_robin: indicates whether sequence p-units regard their scope as circular list.
location: allows to position visual components.
logical_channel: allows to use different (output) devices within one presentation. At presentation time, logical channels are assigned to appropriate physical devices, e.g. displays or loudspeakers. Supports distributed applications.

It depends on the specific realisation of the described synchronisation model, which attributes are supported, whether they are inherited, and on which levels within the document structure they are accepted.

3.2.5 Variables

The author can define variables bound to p-units. They can be set and inquired by directives. They can either be 'private' to the p-unit, or 'public', which makes them visible to other objects according to certain visibility rules. Examples are counters or strings entered by the user.

A special kind of variables are *author-defined signals*. They are controlled by the messages set and unset, and can be used like the predefined signals.

3.3 Directives

Directives are the fundamental tool for specifying additional constraints overriding defaults (Sect. 3.5). A directive describes in its *operation* or *list of operations* (Sect. 3.3.3), what shall be done, and in its *condition* (Sect. 3.3.1), when or while this shall be done. A *condition* is a boolean expression, which leads to the execution of the associated *operation*, as soon as it becomes true, or as long as it is true, depending on the directive's *mode* (Sect. 3.3.2).

3.3.1 Conditions

Conditions serve to describe under which circumstances the operation(s) of a directive shall be executed. They are boolean expressions over signals, states, attributes, and variables. Since these elements always belong to a certain object, usually the addressed object has also to be selected. For the remainder of this paper, the dot-concatenation commonly used in programming languages is used for referencing. For example, X.started denotes the signal started of the object X. And with the usage of the relational operators <, ≤, =, ≠, ≥, >, as well as the boolean operators ∧, ∨, ¬, conditions like

curr_index > 1 ∨ (X.started ∧ (X.state ≠ is_pausing)).

can easiliy be expressed. Furthermore, time offsets can be applied. For example, X.terminated + 2.5 sec denotes a moment in time 2.5 seconds after X emitted terminated.

This results in condition values which may switch between false and true repeatedly during a presentation. (A thorough discussion of this aspect is given in (Herzner and Kummer 1992)). How these switchings control the associated operation(s), depends on the *mode* of the directive.

3.3.2 Modes of Directives

Modes describe how a directive works:

when-mode: the directive executes its operation(s) whenever the condition switches from false to true;

while-mode: the directive executes its operation(s) as long as the condition is true; that means it starts to execute whenever a false→true change occurs, and it terminates the execution whenever a true→false change is encountered.

3.3.3 Operations

Several kinds of operations can be distinguished:

Simple commands: correspond to the messages prepare..stop as shown in Fig. 3.2.

Play commands: perform as long as the condition is true. For example, play X results in a start sent to X at false→true changes of the controlling condition, and in a stop sent to X at opposite turns. They may have initial values for attributes associated, which override defaults.
Furthermore, a while ... pause X behaves analogously.

Modify commands: assign values to attributes or variables, where the values are evaluated in the moment of assignment. If controlled by a while-condition, this results in a continuous update of the target attribute or variable!

A directive may have a list of operations, which are then executed either in parallel or in sequence, depending on the author's specification.

3.4 Input

User input at presentation time is modelled by means of so-called *input objects* adhering to following concepts:

- Several *classes* (Sect. 3.4.1) of input objects are provided.
- For each input class, specific *attributes* describe appearance and behaviour. For example, a 'button' may have attributes describing its shape when inactive, active, or pressed; the conditions for turning to the 'pressed'-state (e.g. 'LeftMouseButtonDown') and back to released, as well as for triggering; and its location and size. And a 'slider' will also have its range as attribute, and perhaps a mapping method from display to value (e.g. linear, logarithmic).
- Each input class provides a signal triggered, which is emitted whenever the user performs a certain action on that input object.
- In addition, most input classes provide a certain attribute reflecting associated user actions, called *measure*.
- Input objects can be driven in one of four *modes* (Sect. 3.4.2).
- Input objects are controlled by the same commands as output objects, and have essentially the same states. For example, a prepared or paused button may be visible, but not usable. However, according to their class, additional signals may be emitted, and further messages may be accepted.

3.4.1 Input Classes

The following classes are considered to be of value in the described environment. However, others are possible or can be derived from existing ones.

Eventer: no own measure. Possible subclasses: buttons, switches, ...
Selector: sequence of alternatives; the measure is the index of the chosen alternative. Possible subclasses: radio button lists, pull down menues, ...
Valuator: the measure is a numerical value. Possible subclasses: sliders, turning knobs, ...
Locator: the measure is a coordinate (pair).
Picker: the measure is (a reference to) a selected object.
String: the measure is a (typed-in or spoken) character sequence.

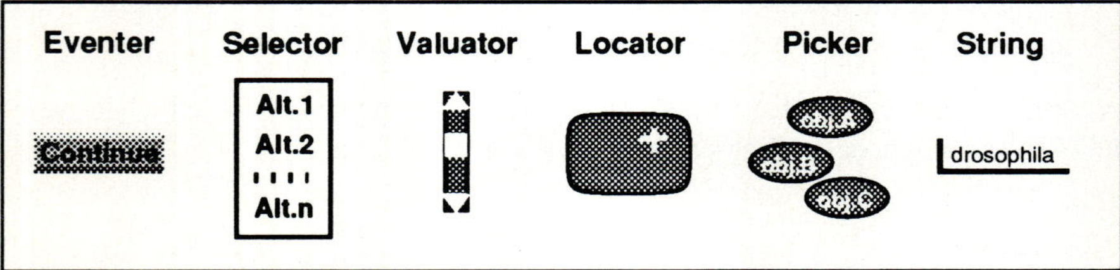

Fig. 3.3. Possible visual presentations of input objects

Note that input classes can also be regarded as sync-types for p-units. Even stronger, when p-units are specified explicitely for input objects, their only valid sync-type is that of the appropriate input class.

Although conventional implementations of such input objects, as depicted in Fig. 3.3, are primarily intended, more sophisticated are not excluded. For example, strings could represent voice input, and in VR (virtual reality) environments, locators could serve for selecting directions, and pickers for grabbing objects. Or eventers could be real hardware like keys on a keyboard.

3.4.2 Input Modes

The mode, a special attribute, selects the general form of interaction:

Single: the signal triggered is released, when the input object is explicitely activated by the user. Then, the input object's state automatically switches to is_pausing; hence, no further input is possible, until it is reset to is_running.

Multiple: like single, but the input object stays in state is_running.

Exclusive: like single, but the whole presentation is paused (except that input object, of course), while the input object is in state is_running. Forces the user to do the requested input; for example, to confirm an error notification.

Continuous: the measure value is continuously updated, without the need of explicit activations by the user. Allows to monitor user actions.

In modes other than continuous, the measure value is updated whenever triggered is released.

3.5 Default Rules

A major objective of the described approach is to ease the author's work as far as possible. For that purpose, the concept of default behaviour is extensively used, making it necessary to specify only those aspects which deviate from default assumptions. (For the explanation of higher and subordinate p-units, see Sect. 3.2.2.)

- An object (p-unit or content-object) begins a life cycle, whenever a higher p-unit (content object) initiates it.
- During a life cycle, an object behaves according to its class (sync-type).
- Directives override default; that means that an object progresses automatically along the life cycle, until it arrives at a state controlled by some directive.

3.5.1 Examples

a) Consider a document, consisting of a sequence of pages, and having the default sync-type sequence. Each page has default sync-type parallel. Then one page will be presented after the other, without having any p-unit defined explicitely.

b) Now, for page 3, a p-unit of class (sync-type) loop is created. Then, it will be shown in a loop, which will be endless, as long as no value for the attribute max_iteration or some input object for termination by the user is provided.

c) Assume that page 3 contains a video V and the input objects Repeat, NextPage of type button as components. A p-unit B shall be defined with the scope (Repeat, NextPage) and the directives

when V.terminated	start B	(1)
when Repeat.triggered	next 3	(2)
when NextPage.triggered	stop 3	(3)

then, per iteration of page 3:

— V starts by default, but Repeat and NextPage don't, because their default behaviour is overridden by B.

— as soon V is terminated, B gets started (1), making Repeat and NextPage available at that time;

— depending on which button is selected by the user, 3 is iterated (2) or terminated (3), the latter causing the presentation to continue with the next page;

— B is terminated when 3 terminates an iteration, because it is subordinate to 3.

4 Realisation

Within the context of Digital's European External Research Program (EERP), a prototype implementation is currently being carried out at Seibersdorf, which finally shall extend CDA (Blake 1990) for the features described in the previous section.

Based on CDA, Digital provides a set of document processing tools like DECpresent (DEC 1990) or DECwrite (DEC 1989). While DECwrite, currently available at least under OpenVMS, ULTRIX, and MS-Windows, initially served for authoring of page-oriented documents, DECpresent is dedicated for the production of colored 'slides', which may both be printed or presented interactively as so-called 'slide-shows'.

Hence, DECpresent has been considered as convenient starting point for a prototype implementation. The presented synchronisation model is mapped to the chosen environment according to the following rules:

- The presentation metaphor is the *slide*. This is a rectangular area which may contain an arbitrary number of content objects, which are either basic output objects or input object.
- Each content, including acoustic clips and input objects, must be contained in some slide.
- For each slide, an arbitrary number of p-units can be defined.
- Each p-unit may comprise nested p-units, whose scopes are subsets of its own scope, and which are completely under its control.
- Directives are always bound to p-units.
- Each slide has the default sync-type parallel, while the document is of sync-type sequence. So, the default presentation behaviour is that of a simple slide show.

During the first phase of the project, which concentrated on the elaboration of the presented synchronisation model, an appropriate scripting language has been specified as well, to support evaluation and testing of the model. Although a graphical ('icon-based') user interface possibly would have been more 'user-friendly', a textual interface was considered to be both easier to specify and implement. Generally, both kinds of user interfaces are considered to be of equivalent power.

4.1 The Script Interface

At most one script can be created per slide, containing all p-units defined for that slide. Here, a p-unit consists of a <header>, which contains

- an optional name for the p-unit,
- the mandatory p-unit class,
- the optional scope: names of components of the slide, where the enumeration defines their ordering,
- an optional list of qualifiers for initializing attributes,

and an optional <body>. User-specific *variables* can be defined here, nested <p-units>, and <directives>. These are like *directives* as described in Sect. 3.3, but with two additions: first, the *condition* is optional, where its omission is equivalent to the condition when true. And, second, *operations* include nested directives. For example, when C1 when C2 P executes P whenever C2 becomes true after C1 has become true.

Within a statement, the name of the p-unit which contains it, can be omitted. In the following, the used grammar is illustrated in a few examples.

4.2 Examples

a) Assume, that some slide contains a text T, a video V, and an audio clip A, where the start-up of V and A may take some time. With a slider S, the user shall be able to control both the volume of A and the size of V (just for demonstration). If T shall be shown immediately, together with some surrogate R for the video, which is displayed until both A and V are prepared, but at least for five seconds, then the following p-unit could be used:

```
parallel                              -- sync-type of the p-unit
  begin                               -- begin of p-unit body
  B: parallel (A, V, S)               -- nested p-unit with name B
    begin
    while is_running                  -- link S' measure to the requested
      begin                           -- attributes, 'relative' means that S' value
      V.sizeX := S.measure relative;  -- is applied as factor to the attr.'s
      V.sizeY := S.measure relative   -- initial value
      A.volume := 10**(S.measure/64) relative;  -- sets volume in dB
      end;                            -- the default mode for sliders is contin.
    when prepared                     -- when B is prepared ...
    and (R.started + 5sec)            -- ... and R shown for 5 seconds, ...
      begin
      start;                          -- ... start B itself and ...
      stop R;                         -- ... stop the surrogate
```

```
      end;
    end;                          -- end of B
  when A.terminated
  and V.terminated stop;          -- stop when both clips have been finished
  end;
```

b) During an exam, the following question should be answered within thirty seconds: "which European states are crossed or bordered by the Danube?" Since the student's knowledge about the names of these states shall be judged, a slide could be created, containing the question at its top, and a matrix of buttons below, each carrying the name of one country. (A further 'start'-button could be provided, but this would give the student time to look after the correct names before clicking on it.) If the student clicked all correct buttons, "ok" shall be displayed, otherwise a "sorry, but the correct states are ...", and all buttons removed which carry names of 'untouched' countries:

```
parallel
  begin
  private signal IsOk, IsWrong;  -- author-defined signals
  Good: parallel                 -- p-unit with correct buttons
        (Austria, .., Romania);
  Bad: parallel                  -- p-unit with wrong buttons
        (Albany, .., UK);
  when (started + 30sec)         -- after 30 seconds ...
    begin
    pause Good, Bad;             -- disable further input,
    when Good.all.triggered
    and not Bad.any.triggered    -- set Ok-signal if only correct buttons
      set IsOk;                  -- have been pressed
    when not Good.all.triggered
    or Bad.any.triggered
      set IsWrong;               -- set Wrong-signal otherwise
    end;
  when IsOk                      -- answer 'ok' when only correct and no
    start Ok;                    -- wrong buttons have been pressed
  when IsWrong
    begin                        -- otherwise,
    start Sorry;                 -- answer 'sorry', and
    stop Bad                     -- remove wrong buttons
    end;
  end;
```

where x.all.y becomes true when all components of x released y, and x.any.y becomes true, when at least one component released y.

c) Finally assume, that several students are tested in parallel with questions like the previous one, while the teacher monitors the progress of the test on their own screen. For that purpose, for each student a window is displayed on the teacher's screen, where results are entered on-line.

To achieve this, for each student a copy of the previous p-unit is made, with an individual name and value for the attribute logical_channel, and having the signals declared with public rather than private. Then, a slide for the monitor windows is created, together with a p-unit describing the required behaviour. It will probably contain statements like

```
when Q7.IsOk     start Question7_Ok;
when Q7.IsWrong  start Question7_Wrong;
```

Finally, for each monitor window, a copy of this p-unit is made, with adapting the referred external names like Q7 to that of the specific student.

5 Conclusion

5.1 Results

A synchronisation model for dynamic documents has been described, which allows for the efficient specification of presentation behaviour in numerous ways:

- Directives provide a powerful and flexible tool to express temporal interdependencies.
- Default behaviour, selected by p-unit classes (sync-types), reduces the author's amount of work.
- P-units and directives support the concept of 'locality'; this not only allows the author to concentrate on local aspects rather than to care about the overall presentation structure all the time, but also eases modifications of 'local' temporal relationships.
- Delays caused by hard- and/or software during presentation time, for example, in distributed environments, can easily be considered.
- An extensive input model allows for various kinds of user interaction with the presentation of documents.
- The application range varies from simple slide shows without dynamic contents to interactive presentations with a variety of dynamic contents and complex synchronisation constraints like computer based training or entertainment.
- Finally, directives provide a means for representing hyper-links.

5.2 Future Work

Undoubtely, there are some aspects related to multimedia documents which are not sufficiently covered by the presented model. So, a first direction for further activities will be that for extending its functionality, where at least the following issues will be addressed:

— Dynamic creation of p-units at presentation time. It is currently not possible to produce an arbitrary number of copies of a certain object (e.g. for presenting it on different screens concurrently), as required in example c) of Sect. 4.2, where the number of students may vary from exam to exam.

— Flexible selection of *scopes* and *operation*-targets. It may sometimes be necessary to select those elements according to different criterions. (For example, all those components of an object which have some attribute set to a certain value or are not input objects.)

— Access to object-specific methods. Consider starting of other applications, or enabling a user to modify a document during presentation; possibly, by adding spoken annotations.

Besides extending the functionality and continuing the implementation, a further topic to be addressed is the comparison with related developments, including international standardisation activities like HyTime (ISO 1992), MHEG (ISO 1993), or PREMO (PRogrammer's Environment for Multimedia Objects). The latter denotes a recently initiated project within ISO/IEC JTC1/SC24, which aims towards an object-oriented system for the (interactive) creation, manipulation and presentation of multimedia information, while MHEG (Multimedia/Hypermedia Expert Group) serves for the coded representation of multimedia information for storage and interchange, also in an object-oriented manner.

For example, MHEG's concept of so-called *presentables* (objects which perform the projection of content objects to perceivable presentations) resemble the *p-units* introduced here. And since MHEG provides a means to attach scripts to objects, it seems to be worthwhile to investigate how the presented approach fits into the MHEG model.

6 Acknowledgements

This work is funded by Digital's European External Research Agreement AU-025A.

The author would like to thank Jack Lenz and Matthias Kummer for their invaluable proofreading.

Authorware Professional is a trademark of Authorware Inc.
DECpresent is a trademark of Digital Equipment Corp.
DECwrite is a trademark of Digital Equipment Corp.
IconAuthor is a trademark of AimTech Corp.
Multimedia Toolbook is a trademark of Asymetrix Corp.
MacroMind Director is a trademark of MacroMind Inc.
OpenVMS is a trademark of Digital Equipment Corp.
ULTRIX is a trademark of Digital Equipment Corp.
MS-Windows is a trademark of Microsoft Corp.

7 References

AimTech Corp. (1992) IconAuthor 4.0 – Reference Manual. Nashua, NH 03063 – 1973, 1992

Asymetrix Corp. (1991) Multimedia Toolbook 1.5. Bellevue, WA 98004, 1991

Authorware Inc. (1992) Authorware Professional Handbook. Berkshire, RG11 6LS, 1992

Blake, J.C., (Ed.) (1990) Compound Document Architecture CDA, Digital Technical Journal Vol.2 No.1. Digital Equip. Corp., Mass., Winter 1990

DEC (1989) DECwrite – User's Guide / Reference Manual. Digital Equip. Corp., Mass.

DEC (1990) DECpresent – User's Guide / Reference Manual. Digital Equip. Corp., Mass.

DEC (1991b) Beyond HyperText: The DECwindows Hyperenvironment Vision. Digital Equipm. Corp., Mass.

Gloor, P.A., Streitz, N.A. (Ed.) (1990) Hypertext und Hypermedia, Informatikfachberichte, Vol.249, Springer 1990

Hahn, B.J., Kahn, P., Riley, V., Coombs, J.H., Meyrowitz, N.K., (1992) IRIS – Hypermedia Services. Communications of the ACM, Vol.35, No.1, pp.36-51, Jan. 1992

Herzner, W., Kummer, M.., (1992) MMV – Synchronizing Multimedia Documents. Proceedings of 2nd Eurographics workshop on Multimedia. Darmstadt 1992, Eurographics Technical Report Series 1992

ISO/IEC (1992) Information Technology – Hypermedia/Time-based Structuring Language (HyTime). ISO/IEC DIS 10744, 1992

ISO/IEC (1993) Information Technology – Coded Representation of Multimedia and Hypermedia Information Objects (MHEG). ISO/IEC CD 13522, 1993

Kummer, M., Kuhn, W., (1991) ASE – Audio and Synchronisation Extension of Compound Documents. Proceedings of 1st Eurographics workshop on Multimedia, Stockholm 1991, Springer EurographicSeminars 1992

MacroMind Inc. (1990) MacroMind Director Version 2.0, User manual. San Francisco, CA 94107, 1990

Petricek, W., Zeiler, M, (1991) Multimedia Database – Computer-aided Education. Informat No.4, pp.6-9, 1991

Yager, T., (1991) Build Multimedia Presentations with MacroMind's MediaMaker. BYTE, pp.302-304, September 1991

Designing Multimedia User Interfaces by Direct Composition

Martin Brenner
Siemens Corporate Research and Development, ZFE ST SN 71,
Otto-Hahn-Ring 6, 81730 München, Germany

Abstract:
A hierarchy of services is needed to support authors and users of multimedia user interfaces. After a short description of this hierarchy, the paper's focus is on the upper levelsof this hierarchy.

This paper recommends the use of the "direct composition" paradigm in multimedia user interface design environments and the benefits of this paradigm are shown.

Finally SX/Tools, a multimedia user interface management system (UIMS) based on direct composition, is described.

1 Author's and User's Needs

1.1 Motivation

In these days the multimedia world is strongly suggestive of the early times of personal computing when every computer progmmer could be quite successful by building and selling self-made word processors. Today not only word processors, but also most of the common application software is standardized and for the economical design of a new application powerful tools are necessary.

Multimedia user interfaces often still are "hand-crafted". But in a few years from now multimedia user interfaces will become widely spread and used and there will be a demand for the design of many different multimedia user interfaces well fit to end-users needs.

To speed up the design of multimedia user interfaces and to minimize the costs for their design powerful tools will be needed to meet multimedia's future challenge.

1.2 Hierarchy of Services

For using and designing multimedia user interfaces a whole hierarchy of services is needed (refer to Fig. 1):

Level 0: Device Drivers

Hardware specific devices are the responsibility of hardware manufactures and therefore only of minor interest for our goalsl.

Level 1: System Services

What is needed for multimedia on the system services level is a (software) platform that minimizes the need for authors to deal with hardware dependencies - as the X window system is a platform for computer graphics. Of course, the author still has to take into account which functionality is available on a specific hardware platform. But it should not be the author's problem *how* to access this functionality.

- Services on the system level should be hardware independent.
- The services should be offered to the user both on local and remote host in the same way.

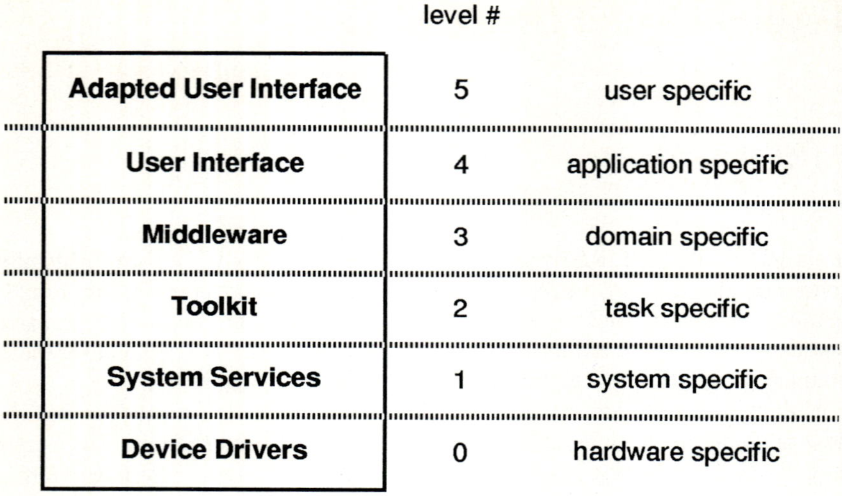

	level #	
Adapted User Interface	5	user specific
User Interface	4	application specific
Middleware	3	domain specific
Toolkit	2	task specific
System Services	1	system specific
Device Drivers	0	hardware specific

Fig. 1: Hierarchy of Services

- These services should include production, presentation, transport across the network, storage and processing of multimedia objects.

Level 2: Toolkit

The toolkit should enable the author to deal with multimedia objects - not with streams of bits and bytes. The toolkit should provide a set of basic multimedia objects and should map the functionality of these basic objects onto the system services mentioned above.
Desired properties of such a toolkit:

- Integration with graphical user interfaces.
  The toolkit should not only provide "office" user interface objects like buttons, menus etc. and multimedia user interface objects, but should also support the design of user interfaces containing graphic user interface objects like circles, polylines, rectangles etc.
- Use of multimedia in the design process.
  The design environment itself should make use of "multimedia" interaction with the designer wherever it is convenient. For example, the help system of the toolkit could provide animated graphics or video clips.
- Openness to new interaction media.
  New interaction media and techniques will appear as well as new tools for interface design coming along with them. In order to avoid "multi-tool" environments which tend to cause severe consistency problems, design environments should be open for a full integration of arbitrary interaction media.
  Again, the use of the new interaction media by the design environment itself should be possible.

- Object-Orientation.
  Each object offers the author all properties changeable in the specific context and all operations executable in the specific context. No additional tool is required to "manipulate" the object.
- The layout of the user interface is designed interactively.
  No programming is needed for specifying layout of a user interface, all can be done fully interactively.
- Dynamic behavior can be defined interactively.
  The interactive behavior of a user interface object is specified by using a script language and by use of spatialization of structure and time. This makes compiling, linking and loading obsolete and allows for very short cycles between design and test.

Level 3: Middleware

Middleware closes the gap between basic objects offered by the toolkit and the author's need of domain-specific sophisticated objects.

Example: Physicians often want to mark an "area of interest" in X-ray images. A new multimedia user interface object has to be built. This object is used in the current design of a user interface and will probably be used in the future design of other interfaces.

The construction of these domain-specific objects should be done by means of the toolkit, not by programming. To achieve this goal some requirements have to be made for the toolkit:

- Aggregation
  The toolkit has to enable the author to combine arbitrary objects to a single, more complex object. Furthermore the author should be able to define interactively the dynamic behavior of the whole object, the dynamic behavior of the parts of the object and the relations between them. In this way the author should be able to define domain-specific objects (or prototypes).
  The author combines a container element, a pixmap and a polyline to a new object of the kind "X-ray image". The author defines: Initially the polyline is invisible. When the user (the doctor) clicks on the image, a visible copy of the polyline is created and the polyline changes according to users mouse movements. In this way no programming was necessary to create an application specific object.
- Design functionality and run-time functionality can be added interactively
  The author adds interactively the functionality for marking areas of interest.
- Support for "Software" Reuse
  The author adds the newly created object "X-ray image" to a domain- specific toolbox. The toolkit should provide support for retrieving other domain specific objects.
- CSCW-Support
  The toolkit should support the construction of a CSCW user interface that allows two or more doctors looking at the X-ray and (visible for their colleagues) marking areas of interest.

Level 4: User Interface

- Availability of design functionality at run time
  Each object has to contain its entire design functionality, which can be used by the end-user, if it is enabled by the author.
  Although the medical doctor as a user is not designing a user interface, he uses the design functionality of the polyline, namely the addition ob points, which was enabled by the author.

- Design functionality as generic application feature
  In user interfaces for some applications the same functionality is necessary as the functionality provided by the design environment at design time.
  For example, when teleconferencing or when using ISDN, users probably want to store, to change, to compose or to pass on drawings, sound, video sequences. Therefore they use the same functionality of multimedia objects as an author.

Level 5: Adaptable User Interface

There is one other reason to put design functionality into the objects themselves:

- Adaptability
  The end-user must be able to adapt application system interfaces for several reasons. First, it is possible to create user-specific interfaces reflecting the personal working style and abilities of individual users.
  Example: About 5% of the male population have problemsin recognizing colors like red or green.
  Second, modification can become necessary when system requirements change and modifications in the structure of the application systems are made. In state-of-the-art automation systems with the ability of dynamic reconfiguration of automation processes this ability to adapt to new application structures is very important.

1.3 Selection of Research Topics

A big part of the multimedia research efforts is concentrated on the lower levels of the services hierarchy, especially on level 0 and level 1. On these levels there is of course still a significant amount of work to be done.

But we expect that within a few years standards for most multimedia data types will be established. It is our goal to be prepared to make use of these standards in a fast, convenient and efficient way - by using tools giving support on the upper levels of the services hierarchy.

2 The Principle of Direct Composition

The term "direct composition" stands for the thorough application of the principle of direct manipulation [4] to the design and development of graphical user interfaces. It characterizes a fully object-oriented approach to the creation and specification of a user interface without using specialized tools. Direct composition is based on an elementary conceptual model of user interface objects [3]. This object model contains both a model of the object's interactive design, and a model of its interactive behavior when using it in the appropriate applicational context (cf. Fig. 2). For this reason each user interface composed of those objects contains a model of its own design and its use.

The static appearance and the interactive behavior of objects described by the conceptual model, which is based on the direct composition philosophy, can be designed by using purely interactive techniques. New objects can be copied or derived from existing ones and both new interface objects and entire user interfaces can be composed directly by using existing objects.

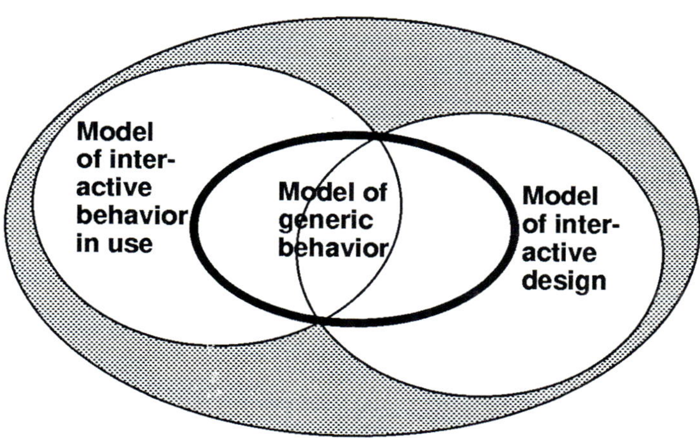

Fig. 2: The object model of direct composition

As a consequence, each object has exactly one set of elementary interaction techniques, one part of which is being used for the dialog with the end-user of a user interface and another, not necessarily disjoint part for the dialog with its designer. The user interface designer can communicate directly with the objects of interest, i.e., with the elements and objects which are combined to form a user interface.The designer does not have to communicate with these objects via separate design tools. The user interface design environment no longer needs to contain tools for dialog design, because all objects of the interface of the design environment and of arbitrary interfaces to be designed contain the means for their own modification and design. Just some browsing facilities should be added to support an easy access to all, even invisible interface objects.

Interface objects define different roles and describe the semantics of the dialog depending on the chosen role. One and the same interaction can cause very different effects on an object according to the role the object takes. The set of interaction techniques of an object includes aspects of manipulation, visualization, and construction. An object always encapsulates the union of all interaction techniques needed in all its roles. The role "design of the object itself", e.g., mainly needs construction aspects, while in the role "dialog with the user of the application" manipulation and visualization aspects usually predominate.

Objects can change their roles and therefore can be used in the design environment as well as in the run-time environment. Moreover, interactive design and testing is not restricted to a specialized design environment but can be activated also at run-time by simply changing the object's role.

To summarize, direct composition of user interfaces offers, among others, the following advantages. Interface objects offer consistent interaction techniques for both the design and usage of user interfaces, end-user adaptability is an inherent feature of direct composition interfaces, and, finally, the openness and extensibility of user interface design systems can easily be achieved by using the compositional approach

3 SX/Tools: A Multimedia User Interface Management System Based On Direct Composition

SX/Tools (S stands for Siemens, X for the X window system) is a homogeneous extensible user interface management system that is designed for the prototyping of complete user interfaces in different application areas.

In the following we describe in how far the requirements stated above are fulfilled by this UIMS. It is shown that direct composition plays a major role in meeting many of these requirements.

3.1 The layout of the user interface is designed interactively

SX/Tools follows the principle of direct composition as described above. Each interface object contains all the knowledge necessary for its own design and for its use as part of an application interface.

With SX/Tools, interfaces are built by copying and modifying existing interface components and creating new components by composition of basic elements. The interaction process for the design follows a direct manipulation style, i.e., the designer does not have to write code in order to define a user interface, but, instead, can concentrate on the ergonomic features of the user interfaces to be designed.

Properties which can be modified by direct manipulation (e.g., size, position, rotation) can be defined either using a pointing device or like all other properties using property sheets. The principle of direct composition applies to those other properties, too. Each property knows how it can be modified in an optimal way from the user's point of view and uses an appropriate property sheet for its design. These property sheets can also be adapted to specific hard- and software requirements. and to users's preferences

3.2 Integration with graphical user interfaces

SX/Tools handles rectangular "form" objects (buttons, menus...), arbitrary graphics (lines, polygons, raster images...) and multimedia objects in a homogeneous manner. These objects can be arbitrarily combined in a user interface.

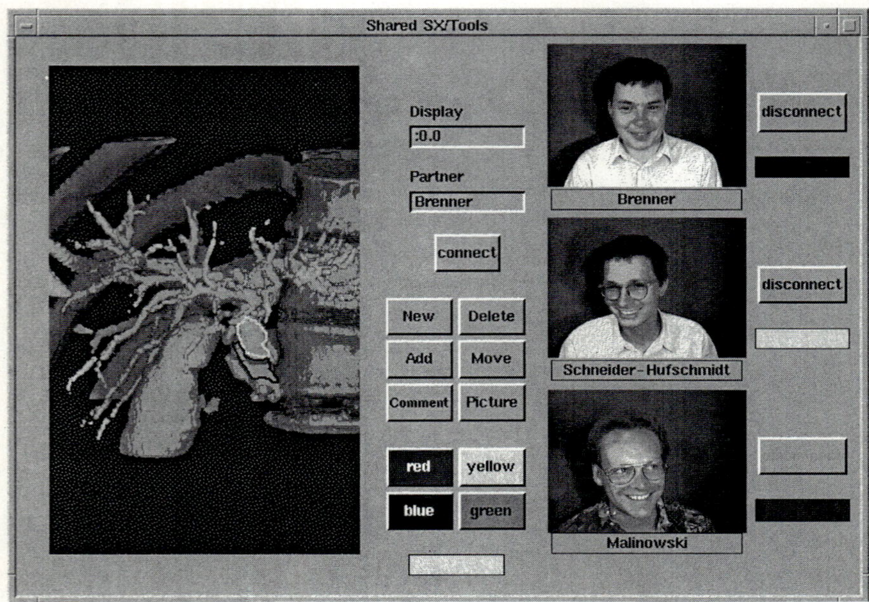

cation (currently showing Siemens UI-researchers)

Fig. 3 shows a prototypical user interface for a medical CSCW - application allowing doctors at different remote places to mark areas of interest in a X-ray image and making voice annotations to their marks. In this user interface form objects, like buttons, graphics objects like polylines, and multimedia objects like pixmaps and sound data are combined.

3.3 Openness to new interaction media

X/Tools is an open user interface design environment. The integration of new interaction media is relatively simple. Although some programming effort is necessary the integration of audio or video output on a given platform is not a major problem.

Extensions to SX/Tools can be obtained through further development of basic toolboxes by adding new, interactively designed interaction techniques. Only the most basic techniques (e.g., the handling of new i/o channels) have to be implemented by conventional object-oriented, programming. Internally such elementary techniques are encapsulated in classes. Prototypical Instances of these classes are used as toolbox representations.

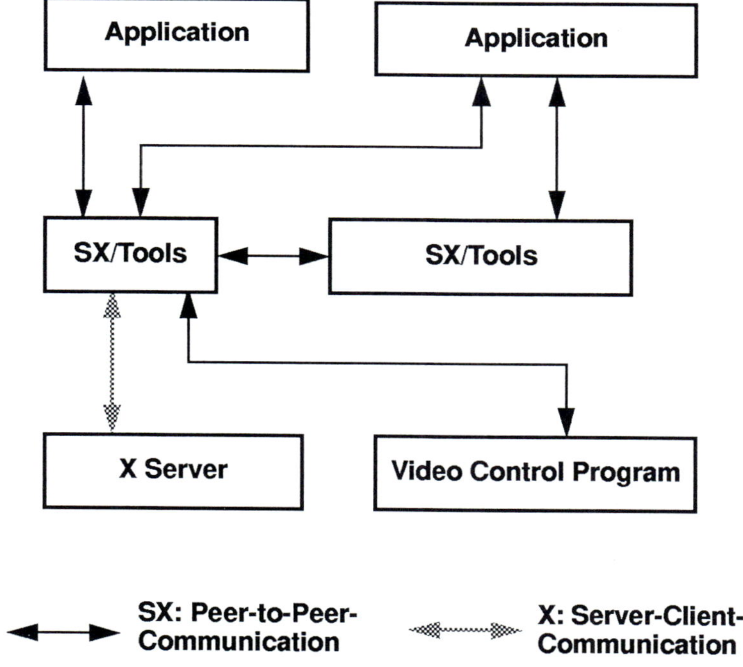

Fig. 4: Using the SX/Tools Peer-to-Peer communications for integration of video functionality

Alternatively, SX/Tools Peer-to-Peer - Communications Features can be used for integrating new media support.

Certainly, more effort is needed to really integrate these interaction media, but the experiences so far have been encouraging.

3.4 Use of multimedia in the design process

The *openness* of the user interface management system extends into the design of the UIMS itself. The designer is free to define some personal environment in which the further use of SX/Tools is performed. The use of domain specific toolboxes containing interactive graphical elements and layout elements is just one example for this possibility. Since each object in a direct composition environment contains the information necessary for its own design and use, the same is true for the elements comprising the design environment. This property has the consequence that after the realization of the basic elements of the UIMS (the "bootstrapping phase"), the entire system can be developed using its own design techniques. Tools necessary in the UIMS for the design of interfaces can be designed in the same way as the interfaces themselves.

3.5 Object-Orientation

There is no need for separate tools in the design environment since every SX/Tools object contains the functionality for both its design and usage.

Therefore, in SX/Tools there is no separation between runtime and design environment. This gives the possibility of using design functionality at run-time either as feature of the user interface or for user interface adaptation by the end-user or by the system [2].

A second important advantage of the uniformity of design and runtime environment is the ability to switch between design and simulation "on the fly". This allows for very rapid repetitions of "design - test" - cycles.

3.6 Dynamic behavior can be defined interactively

For the definition of dynamic properties of user interfaces (the "behavior") different techniques have been proposed, among the most commonly used are state-transition-nets, context-free grammars and event-based techniques. For a discussion of the advantages and disadvantages of these approaches we refer to Green [3]. For the development of SX/Tools we have chosen an event-based approach. One of the advantages of this approach is that the reaction to incoming events can be defined locally at the user interface objects conforming to the principle of object-orientation. The overall behavior of the user interface can then be described by the interplay of the local reactions to incoming events.

For the description of the reaction to incoming events (called scripts) a simple C-like language SX/Talk has been defined. To relieve the user interface designer from the burden of knowing the syntax of this language exactly, SX/Tools provides an interactive, structure-oriented editor for event-definitions. This can again be seen as an example of direct composition: if the designer wants to define a script of an object a specific modification tool is instantiated to perform the task for that object. The reaction to an incoming event can be either the modification of local properties, the application of other local scripts or the creation of an event being sent to another object of the user interface or the application system. Scripts are not compiled and linked into the UIMS-code. Scripts are parsed and a syntax check is performed on their contents. Afterwards, a binary version of scripts becomes a property of the user interface object in question. This version of the scripts is then interpreted. The reason for this solution is that the user interface need not be compiled and linked after each modification (see above).

Events may be either system-defined or user-defined. System-defined events include mouse-clicks, key-presses and selections in menus. User-defined events can be of any kind. These events are sent to interface objects either from the application system or from other user interface objects.

3.7 Aggregation

Aggregation can be done without explicitly writing code. Existing objects are copied and combined into new objects, so-called aggregate objects. These objects behave like simple objects. They also have static properties which define their appearance and it is possible to define scripts which control their behavior. Aggregate objects can be copied into toolboxes and be made available for future use.

As illustrated by Fig. 5, the direct composition approach implies a uniform interface development process which covers tool development, interface design and "on-usage" interface adaptation. The entire process is performed within one and the same environment following the same basic principles. This is in contrast to the conventional approach of separated design and runtime environments [5] found in most state-of-the-art UIMSs.

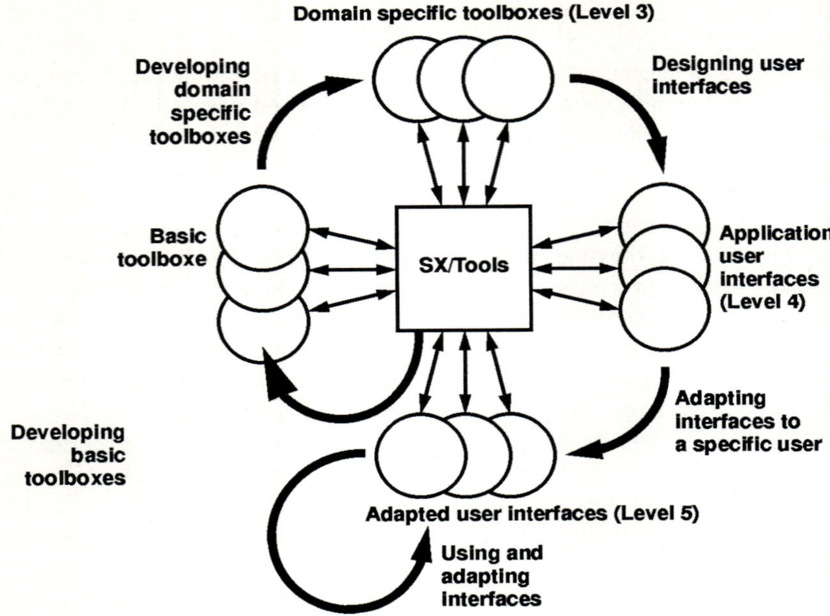

Fig. 5: The SX/Tools interface development process

3.8 Support for Software Reuse

Interface components can be collected into so-called toolboxes. Basic toolboxes exist, e.g., for graphics, forms, windows, menus, multimedia etc. New toolboxes can be created in the same way as new interfaces, namely by interactively copying objects from other toolboxes or interface definitions. Toolboxes as well as interfaces can be stored permanently and their contents can be used in later sessions. According to the principle of direct composition, the necessary object management is performed by each object itself.

3.9 Adaptability

Objects in direct composition environments like SX/Tools contain the information about their modification *and* their use. These two parts usually cannot be separated easily. Therefore interfaces designed with SX/Tools contain the possibility for their own modification even after the delivery to the end-user. The user of an application system can modify its user interface using the same techniques and tools as the designer. The interaction techniques employed during the modification of user interface components are the same that the user knows from the interaction with the application system itself.

3.10 availability of design functionality at run time / design functionality as generic application feature

Because all objects contain the information about their modification, this design functionality can be used as a feature of the user interface at run time.

3.11 design functionality and run-time functionality can be added interactively

The customization of the design environment can easily be accomplished by interactive development of domain specific toolboxes. Fig. 6, e.g., shows toolboxes designed for interface construction in the domain of business graphics, traffic management systems and a toolbox with objects supporting some CSCW (Computer Supported Cooperative Work) functions. Domain specific toolboxes provide the user interface designer with elements which fit the application's needs through an adequate level of abstraction.

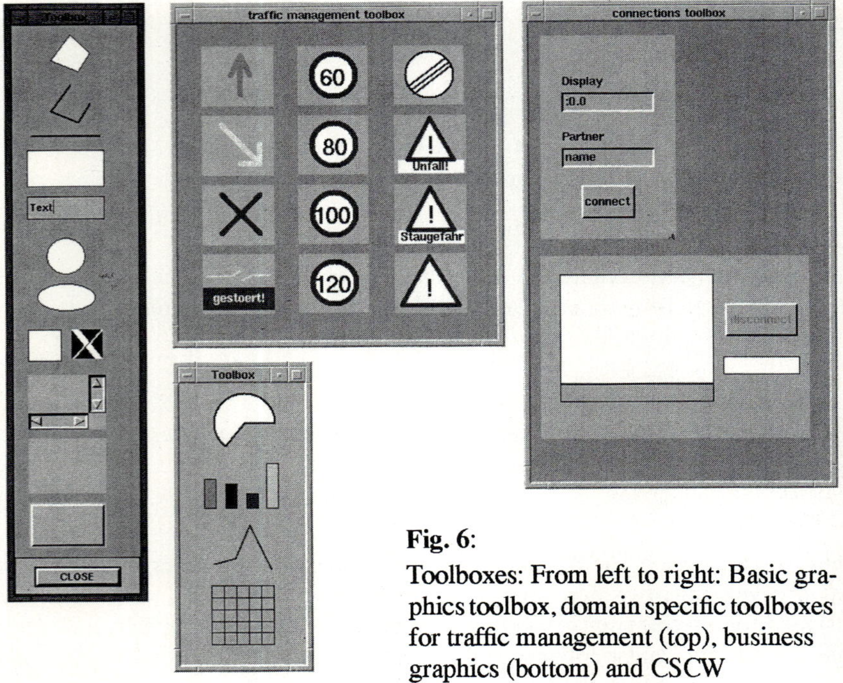

Fig. 6:

Toolboxes: From left to right: Basic graphics toolbox, domain specific toolboxes for traffic management (top), business graphics (bottom) and CSCW

3.12 CSCW-Support

SX/Tools has been designed with a client-server structure. Each SX server can interact with an arbitrary number of application systems and an application system can cooperate with many SX servers. This allows for both large applications being controlled from several workstations and one workstation controlling many small applications.

Furthermore two or more SX servers can communicate with each other ("*peer-to-peer-communication*"). Objects on local and remote peers can be addressed in a homogenous way. This enables the author to design CSCW supporting user interface with SX/Tools. Refer to Fig. 3 for a user interface supporting CSCW made with SX/Tools.

Addressing of a object on the local peer:

```
"myobjectname".do_it (arg1,arg2,arg3);
```

Addressing of an object on a remote peer:

```
@"Peer":"myobjectname".do_it (arg1,ar-
```

Fig. 7: Example for addressing local and remote objects

3.13 State of the SX/Tools Implementation

A prototype of the SX/Tools user interface management system has been implemented. The system has been used for the design of protoypes of user interfaces for automation systems and process control systems. A product version for the design of graphical user interfaces (without multimedia objects) is planned for summer ´93.

Current work covers the further integration of multimedia and multimodal techniques. The next steps in the development of SX/Tools may include improvements on level 4 ("user interface") by adding a application model support and on level 5 ("adapted user interface") by adding features for the support of adaptive user interfaces.

4 Concluding Remarks

This paper has attempted to point out some markedly important requirements of multimedia user interface management. In particular, the growing variety of interaction media and techniques as well as the current trend to a higher degree of end-user participation in the design process of user interfaces have to be taken into account. The support of the user interface author will gain in significance as use and design of multimedia user interfaces will become routine. Thus, a model is needed that covers the aspects of the upper levels services hierarchy of complex interfaces, but, on the other hand, is as simple as possible.

The principle of direct composition is considered to be such a simple design model which can serve as a basis for appropriate architectures of multimedia user interface design environments.

4.1 Acknowledgements

Portions of this paper were taken from [1] and [2]. I am very grateful to Matthias Schneider-Hufschmidt, Thomas Kühme and Daniel Aliaga, the authors of these reports, for their contributions to this paper. For the final version of this paper I got valuable hints from Matthias Schneider-Hufschmidt and Uwe Malinowski.

4.2 References

1. Kühme, Th., Schneider-Hufschmidt, M. *SX/Tools - An Open Design Environment for Adaptable Multimedia User Interfaces* in: Alistair Kilgour, Lars Kjelldahl (Eds.): *Eurographics '92, Proceedings of the European Computer Graphics Conference*, Computer Graphics Forum, Vol. 11, Nr. 3, Cambridge, UK.pp. C-93 - C-105, NCC Blackwell Publishers, Oxford.

2. Daniel Aliaga, Matthias Schneider-Hufschmidt P*rototyping of Graphing Tools by Direct GUI Composition - an Experience Report*, to be published in: *Proceedings of the RE ´93*, Bonn.

3. Kühme, Th., Hornung, G. and Witschital, P. *Conceptual models in the design process of direct manipulation user interfaces.* In: H.-J. Bullinger (ed.): *Human Aspects in Computing: Design and Use of Interactive Systems and Work with Terminals.* Proceedings of the HCI International '91, Stuttgart, F.R.G., Elsevier, 1991, pp. 722-727.

4. Shneiderman, Ben. *Direct Manipulation: A Step Beyond Programming Languages*, IEEE Computer 16, 8 (August 1983), pp. 57-69.

5. Green, M. *Report on Dialogue Specification Techniques.* In: [6], pp. 9-20.

6. Pfaff, Günther E. (ed.). U*ser Interface Management Systems.* Proceedings of the Workshop on User Interface Management Systems held in Seeheim, FRG, November 1-3, 1983, Springer, Berlin, 1985.

7 ... other papers referred to the workshop

Using Conceptual Maps in Hypermedia

Jerker J. E. Andersson
Infologics, P.O. Box 91, S-191 22 Sollentuna, Sweden
WM-data Education, P.O. Box 27030, S-102 51 Stockholm, Sweden

1 Hypertext and Hypermedia

In the field of hypertext and hypermedia there is an on-going discussion concerning link and node-models [2, 6, 10, 14]. There have been some systems that have explicitly separated structure and content, e.g. Intermedia's concept of "webs" being superimposed on "documents" [6, 17].

There are different notions of what a link is and what a node is [2, 4, 15]. There are also different ideas of what a hypermedia anchor is. There are structured links that could very well become nodes in their own right, as been done in Notecards [3]. Other argue that a link should have no properties at all, like in KMS. There are also several suggestions for database-like hyperspaces that support typed links and nodes [11, 15].

There is also a recognized need for supporting the user in forming a mental model of the hyperspace. This can be done by providing different tools and access points suitable for different information retrieval situations. Providing the right mechanisms for selection and feedback has been identified as a very important factor for hypermedia usability [13, 15].

2 The Overview Problem

This well known problem [2] have attracted a lot of attention. To make a long story short: The potential connectivity in a multidimensional information space provides endless opportunities for searching and therefore also for getting lost. If the relation between bits of information is not clear, the user's view becomes fragmented, making it difficult to develop a feeling of 'here' (instead it might become a feeling of 'where am I?')

This leads to several problem situations: Firstly, the user might not be able to find his or her way back to some information that he or she has seen before. Also, the user cannot make an effective plan of how to search for something new. And, even worse, he or she may not know if the search is exhaustive, has all relevant information been found? All this leads to frustration and the possibility that the hypermedia system is less effective than a conventional information system [15].

3 Previously Proposed Improvements

There are numerous supportive functions and strategies that could prove helpful in battling the navigation problem. The nature of each multimedia information system, as well as it's users goals and motives, is unique. Hence the remedies for curing the navigation problem and their effectiveness vary from case to case.

To start with we should note that traditional media is full of supporting functions and guiding information. These have been worked out by skilful writers and designers during hundreds of years (maybe just a single hundred for moving images, still a fair amount of time). They are integrated into our culture and are sometimes so subtle that they are noticed only when absent.

Computer based multimedia can be considered a new media [10] (there are other 'multimedias' beside the computer based one) and has very little user experience to build upon. It makes use of interactions and has a discrete structure. The information is often cut into little pieces, called *nodes*, to be *linked* together again in a flow chart, a tree, a web or a similar structure. The structure is then *navigated* by a user employing *navigation tools*. Here follows a few of the proposed mechanisms used for browsing hypermedia [2, 7, 15]:

Guided tours (or super links) that steps through a number of nodes serves to show the structure of the system and how it's functions can be used. *Back-tracking* provides a general function for retracing one's own steps to try another approach. *History list* is a 'visible' back-tracking mechanism, simply select how far back you want to go. They can be more or less graphical. *Maps* or *diagrams* are helpful in real life and why not in 'hyperspace'. The problem is that screen-space only allows for a few nodes and links to be shown at one time. The 'cartographer' may design different maps for different user/problem categories. Then we have *zooming* and *scrolling* devices such as fish-eye views, scrolling walls [12] or folding structures (such as in-line expansion of text, the folders of the Macintosh Finder or the cone-trees and can-trees conceived by Xerox PARC [16]).

But a designer can also make use of traditional knowledge about information structuring: Indexing and key-word extraction are two examples. Also, since we are using traditional media as building blocks we have their tool-boxes available as well: run in references, picture focussing, parallel actions used in films, external story teller and much more [10]. And finally a user could always ask the next user down the LAN.

To expand a little on the ideas of using maps, one can say that complete maps of a hyperspace are unmanageable at best [2] and typically to large to be useful. For a meaningful number of nodes, screen-space is quickly consumed. The first fix to the screen-space problem is a hierarchical map, showing increasing levels of details as one selects nodes, going downward. Once again the context is lost when higher levels are no longer visible. Other forms of adapting graphs have been proposed with good results [5], where the user retains some context from all levels that are "above " the current level. Knowledge of how to design graphics interfaces can also be used to provide some stable elements on screen that support the context. One example is to employ the lexivisual structures that are used in comics [9]

4 Our Proposal: Use the Inherent Structure of the Domain to Provide a Conceptual Map

In order to do as much as possible with the screen-space available we tried another approach on the map/diagram solution. Why not use the inherent structure in a domain to get a semi-organised categorisation of the information? This would then be used to label the information and to provide a *conceptual map*. This map tool would allow browsing by selecting a group of nodes associated by their categorisation and relation to the current node. From this subset the user then selects his next destination node.

This is how we propose to elicit such inherent structures; Experts of the domain could participate in a conceptual analysis. This would provide a set of concepts used for categorising information in a domain (example for a sales-mans application could be: component, product, product family, technical description, sales description, example of use and price-list). The relations between these concepts could be found at the same time. The result would be something similar to a conventional database model, but far less formal.

Each node in the hypermedia system would get a label that put it in a category (as wide or narrow definition as the domain experts require). At the same time the relations to other concepts would provide a basic set of structural links to neighbouring nodes. More links could be added by the author in traditional hypermedia manner for references or associations not covered by the general model.

4.1 A Screen Layout Example

The main area in figure 4.1 is the view area were the subject content is displayed (text, graphics, still picture etc). The top right window is a navigation tool displaying a history list. The middle right window contains the conceptual map, further described below. The bottom right window is an alphabetical index and the wide window at the bottom is a hierarchical table of contents.

When running the system, one window displays a map based on the conceptual model (middle right window in figure 4.1). When a concept (blob) in the map is clicked at, it pops up a list of all entries in the corresponding category. The user makes a selection or clicks at another concept to see another list. At all times the 'current' concept is highlighted corresponding to the category of the 'current' node (the last selected or topmost piece of information shown in the main area).

If the user follows an associative link in, say a in picture, by selecting something in it directly, the context may change radically. The user wouldn't know if he or she made a small move locally or jumped to the other end of the 'hyperspace'. But if the map of the conceptual model is present it would highlight the appropriate concept showing how far the jump was in that aspect.

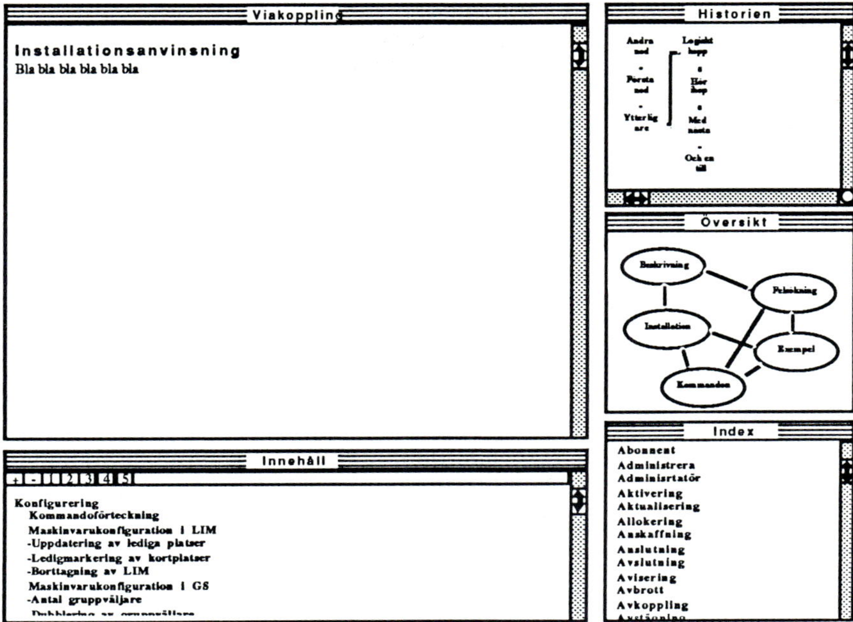

Fig. 4.1 Example of screen layout with four navigation tools.

Another feature that can be used is the 'selective category'. Imagine that a salesman is reviewing a component description. When he selects the product concept the system could use the link information to show only the products using that particular component. Of course, if he so desires, the full list of all products can be displayed as an alternative.

5 A Mechanism for Managing Information and Meta-Information to Generate the Conceptual Map

The conceptual map tool as envisaged could be a generic tools. That means that if we change the model, the number of concepts or relations, or if we edit our actual data content the changes are reflected automatically in the map tool's aspect and behaviour. The dynamics thus required can be achieved by a de-coupling of the structural information from the content data.

In doing so we can sift and rearrange nodes by comparing their relations to each other and looking at their attributes, i.e. labels. If this information is maintained in a separate index we do not need to parse the content of nodes. We simply issue a query corresponding to the current context and the users action. A side effect is that such an index can be used for supporting a number of navigation tools. Thus allowing us a greater amount of freedom when design our users environment.

Several such models, providing a de-coupling of content and structure, have been proposed within research literature and it will not be addressed further in this context. In figure 5.1 below is a schematic drawing of the underlaying mechanism we used, called HAM, Hypermedia Abstract Machine.

It handles the information to support the conceptual map tool [1]. As was mentioned above it is a generalized model to support any tool the user would like to have. A de-coupling of the navigation from the content is reached through providing a separate index, the conceptual model, that contains information about the arrangement of the actual subject matter (in the media boxes at the bottom).

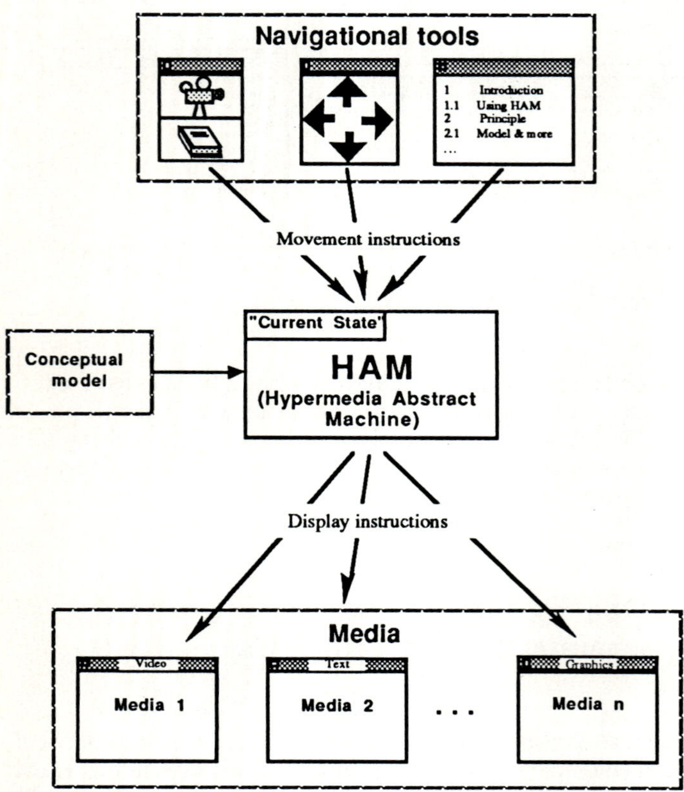

Fig. 5.1 Functional view of the HAM

5.1 HAM modus operandi

The central part is the actual HAM engine that coordinates and evaluate the users action in order to decide where the user moves and what nodes to show. It stores the current state, can evaluate relative movement and absolute addresses and acts as an information server for the other parts. In order to map node-names onto granules it has got an index. It list nodes by names and show what media they contain. The index also contains domain topological information such as arrangement of the nodes into chapters and sub-chapters.

Next there is the top layer in the graph. The user can interact with a number of different navigation tools, some of which might be custom built for a particular user group or presentation. We have designed a minimal set of generic tools such as the browsing arrows moving forward or backward, topic selections lists and a media selection palette. These, and any other tool we might design, employ a simple language to tell the HAM what actions the user has taken. The HAM in it's turn evaluates what effect that action will have on the current state and issues commands accordingly. We have conducted some experiments using custom built tools to annotate and save "trails" which we will discuss further later on.

Lastly we have the media managers that takes care of retrieval from the various media databases as well as displaying and searching in the different media. Each media manager has display methods and search methods to obey the commands of the HAM engine. A video manager, for instance, knows where to find a particular sequence demanded by the HAM and how to display it in a designated window. The window might be freely movable by the user or under the control of some navigation tool.

6 Experiment and Evaluation Method Employed

In evaluating the usability of the conceptual map tool we performed a user study at TELI, a Swedish company [8]. An electronic manual covering part of a computerized telephone exchange was used for the experiment. It was produced in the manner described above in cooperation with domain expertise and information modelling expertise.

The test group consisted of six technicians using computers and window based applications daily but with no prior experience with this type of systems. Some were knowledgeable in the subject domain and had previous experience of the paper based counterpart of the electronic manual.

A set of tasks were prepared by the domain expertise, all well within the regular problem domain of the manual provided. The subjects were confronted with the system individually. They were told to describe their understanding of the concepts in the map and to draw another map of their own using a super-set of concepts. The various navigations tools of the system were described and the subjects were told to solve the tasks and put down the results on paper.

All actions were logged and the subjects were encouraged to 'think aloud' and their comments were taped.

7 Results from the Evaluation Experiment

The results of the study were meant to indicate whether or not further work on this specific tool would be of interest. The small group of subjects and the short time and reduced scope of the evaluation experiment severely limits the usefulness of the results. We would argue, however, that the findings at least warrants a closer look at the possibilities at hand.

In the time allowed, all subjects solved one or more problems, all problems pursued were answered correctly. The distribution of use of the navigation tools is shown in figure 7.1. The preferred means of navigation was the 'regular' hypermedia links, closely followed by the history list tool and the conceptual map tool. The index was used less frequently.

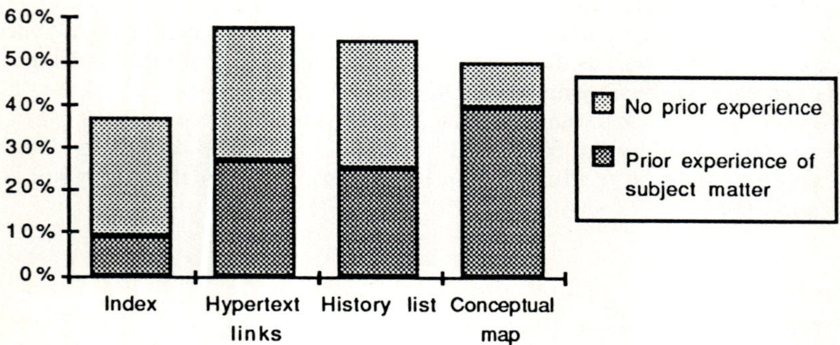

Fig. 7.1 Aggregation of mean use of types of navigation for the two groups.

The most significant observation to be made was that the subjects with some prior knowledge of the subject matter from conventional manuals used the conceptual map more frequently. The probable reason for this would be familiarity with the concepts and hence a willingness to use them. The users that were unfamiliar with the domain relied on more traditional methods, having a notably higher use of the conventional index.

8 Pitfalls

Do not design a database. The experts may propose too detailed concepts or attributes or relations with qualifiers. If you want a database, that should have been clear earlier on.

Be careful in selecting concepts. Experts seldom agree. Which one is right? The users don't care for theoretical aspects. If they don't understand the concepts the system won't work for them. Either select other concepts or educate the users. Many times the dialogue between the domain experts and the users shows that the problem of understanding may well lie with the communication between groups rather than between man and machine. Try having the users label examples selecting from the experts vocabulary to see were they agree and disagree. This area is subject to research within information and business modelling.

Make sure the intended users have some training in using the map-tool and understand the concepts. The intuitive aspects of user interfaces are important but in professional systems walk-up-and-use interfaces quickly become cumbersome. Therefore we would recommend designing for the user that has become familiar with the system and invest in educating the novice user to achieve some level of expertise.

9 Conclusions

The use of conceptual models and an associated map tool can be helpful in navigating a multimedia application. This is especially true in semi-structured domains such as manuals, technical handbooks and similar professional productions. Such a tool can also be generic and thus support a dynamic hypermedia information system.

The success of a conceptual map tool also depends on how well the end-user understand the concepts the experts of the domain are using. Therefore, research and experiences from information and business modelling will be important as pointed out above. Much work can also be done in comparing different sets of concepts. Other research is needed in comparing different set of navigation tools and their learning curve as well as the relative importance of structural and associative links.

Acknowledgements

The author wish to thank Peter Rosengren, originator of the conceptual maps, for his never ending support and constant flow of brilliant ideas. Also many thanks to Dr. Cecilia Katzeff for her work and contributions, both working at SISU, Swedish Institute for Systems Development in Kista, Sweden.

References

1 Jerker Andersson, "A Design Proposal for a Hypermedia Abstract Machine" in Multimedia: Systems, Interaction and Applications, L. Kjelldahl (Ed.), Springer Verlag, 1992

2 Jeff Conklin, "Hypertext: An Introduction and Survey", IEEE Computer September, 1987

3 Frank Halasz, "Reflections on Notecards: Seven Issues for the Next Generation of Hypermedia Systems", Communications of the ACM, July 1988

4 Frank Halasz & Jeff Conklin, "Issues in the Design and Application of Hypermedia Systems", Tutorial CHI 90, ACM New York, 1990

5 Tyson R. Henry, Scott E. Hudson, "Interactive Graph Layout", Proc of ACM/UIST 1991, ACM New York, 1991

6 Matthew E. Hodges, Russell M. Sasnett & V. Judson Harward, "Musings on Multimedia", Unix Review Vol 8 No 2, 1990

7 Cecilia Katzeff, "The Overview Problem in Hypermedia - a Congnitive Perspective", Report in Swedish, SISU-rapport no. 18, SISU, PO Box 1250, 164 28 Kista, Sweden, 1992

8 Cecilia Katzeff, "Report from a Study of Users of Electronic Manuals at Teli", Report in Swedish, In print, SISU, PO Box 1250, 164 28 Kista, Sweden, 1992

9 Mikael Kindborg, "Visual Techniques for Orientation in Hypermedia Structures", Licentiate Thesis, Dep. of Computer & Systems Science, University of Stockholm/ Royal Institute of Technology, Sweden, 1991

10 Brenda Laurel, Tim Oren & Abbe Don, "Issues in Multimedia Interface Design: Media Integration and Interface Agents", Proc of ACM/SIGCHI 90, ACM New York, 1990

11 Jesper Lundh, "Data Models in Hypertext", SISU, Box 1250, S-164 28 Kista, Sweden, 1989

12 Jock D. Mackinlay, George G. Robertson, Stuart K. Card, "The Perspective Wall: Detail and Context Smoothly Integrated", Proc of ACM/SIGCHI 91, ACM New York, 1991

13 Gary Marchionini & Ben Shneiderman, "Finding Facts vs. Browsing Knowledge in Hypertext Systems", IEEE Computer January, 1988

14 Norman Meyrowitz, "The Link to Tomorrow", Unix Review vol 8 no 2, 1990

15 Jacob Nielsen, "Hypertext and Hypermedia", Academic Press 1990

16 George G. Robertson, Jock D. Mackinlay, Stuart K. Card, "Cone Trees: Animated 3D Visualization of Hierarchical Information", Proc of ACM/SIGCHI 91, ACM New York, 1991

17 Nicole Yankelovich et al, "Intermedia: The Concept and the Construction of a Seamless Information Environment", IEEE Computer January, 1988

Word and Image in Multimedia

Jay David Bolter and Kenneth J. Knoespel
School of Literature, Communication, and Culture &
Graphics, Visualization and Usability Laboratory
LCC-0165, Georgia Institute of Technology, Atlanta, GA, USA 30332-0165

Rhetoric is an ancient term that is not often thought relevant to the contemporary world of electronic communication. For thousands of years, rhetoric has been defined as the art of writing or speaking persuasively, and so has been limited to verbal communication. But even in the age of printed books, effective communication has often included pictures and graphs as well as words. Computer-controlled multimedia, which is a new form of communication, goes further and includes animated graphics, sound, and video. At the technical level, standards for storing, compressing, and representing text, graphics, and video are being defined: standards such as RTF, SGML, Quicktime, JPEG, MPEG, ODA, HyTime, and MHEG. (See for example 2992, HyT92, and ODA89). But at the level of presentation and interaction in multimedia environments, a different kind of standard must be developed. For these new media require that we expand our definition of rhetoric. We must define a rhetoric of multimedia: a set of design rules and practices that suggest how to create persuasive combinations of all the media mentioned above.

Together with colleagues in the School of Literature, Communication, and Culture and the Graphics, Visualization, and Usability Center at the Georgia Institute of Technology, we are working to establish the rudiments of a such rhetoric.[1] Our goal is to explore effective configurations of old and new media. We want to learn how to draw on classical rhetorical theory and the history of writing to improve current multimedia design. And we want to see whether current theories of art, music, and literature can help us understand multimedia. (See, for example, Laurel91.) We believe that these historical and theoretical

---

1 We must think beyond a rhetoric of multimedia that pertains only to the commercial applications of computer technology. We find ourselves developing an integrative theory that follows decades of work that had questioned the status of text and image. At a time when we have learned to destabilize virtually any text or image through skeptical methodologies, multimedia challenges us to ask how the critical work of the past years may come to bear on electronic technologies. The development of a rhetoric of multimedia would provide a set of critical perspectives for improving multimedia presentations. The definition of such perspectives would rely on the understanding that rhetoric, even as classically defined, is an integrative practice including the graphic and aural. Multimedia challenges us to see how flattened or two dimensional our means of communication have become. Finally, the definition and practice of a rhetoric of multimedia would depend on the integration of art history and musicology with literary theory. Colleagues in the School of Literature, Communication, and Culture at Georgia Tech who have participated in the discussions regarding the development of a rhetoric of multimedia include Professors Anne Balsamo, Charles Bazerman, Peter McGuire, and Stuart Moulthrop.

considerations can and should be combined with experience in computer graphics, human-computer interface design, and other disciplines in computer science.

In this paper we offer an example of our interdisciplinary approach to the rhetoric of multimedia. We consider the problem of integrating verbal texts into graphic environments, a problem that has received relatively little attention. Designers of multimedia applications tend to emphasize graphics and particularly video. When used at all, text is relegated to a separate space, often in a separate window. There are historical reasons for the separation of text and graphics in multimedia. Computer text processing developed earlier and in a separate tradition from computer graphics. Word processors in personal computers are about a decade old; business word processors were already common in the 1970s, and text editors for programming in time-shared mainframes date from the 1960s. The early generations of word processors were of course wholly alphanumeric. Advances in hardware and software have made possible first bitmapped graphics and then computer-generated animation and computer-controlled video and sound. These advances have led to new applications, but these new applications have little use of text beyond the obvious need to make labels. We still have largely discrete sets of applications for text (databases, word processors) and for graphics and video (image processing, multimedia presentations).

Although this division may have been appropriate in the past, a number of forces are driving us toward integration. As the hardware and software for digitizing and storing images becomes less expensive, users are expecting to be able to include graphics in their documents and presentations. Multimedia databases of archives materials (e.g. newspaper articles together with their photographs) now become thinkable. Encyclopedias (e.g. Grolier's Electronic Encyclopedia) are beginning to include pictures and even sound. Soon video will be included in such products. In the first such applications it may just be a matter of opening a window and showing the graphic or video. But in the long run, we need to rethink how words and images can share the same visual and conceptual space in the computer.

To help in this process of rethinking, we propose to look back into the history of the printed book. Printers confronted similar issues in the first three hundred years of their technology, as they slowly learned how to arrange words spatially to convey structure and meaning and how to add graphics (woodcuts and then copper engravings) to the stream of words. The art of typography developed into a sophisticated set of practices between the 1450s and 1700. Studying these practices can help us define a new "typography" for the space provided of computer-controlled multimedia.

1. Spatial Text in Earlier Print Technology

The printing press was invented in the middle of the fifteenth century, and at first printed books were made to look very much like fifteenth-century manuscripts. The process of making the books changed, but the product remained almost the same. [Eisenstein1979, pp. 51-52.] This similarity was natural: printers wanted to sell their books to readers who were used to manuscripts. Furthermore, printers themselves did not immediately see any need to change the form of the book: they were accustomed to the (German) manuscript's dark pages of Gothic script. Over the next several generations, books did change. But even in the sixteenth century they retained some of the organizational and visual characteristics of the medieval manuscript. For example, as in medieval manuscripts, many older texts (particularly Greek and Latin authors and legal works) continued to be printed with commentaries, and these commentaries were sometimes layed out around the original text in layers. The printed page was divided into zones: the texts in the outer zones explained the text in the center.

A good example is provided by this standard edition of the Latin poet Ovid's Metamorphoses, published in 1565. (See figure 1.) Ovid's poem itself is located in the center in a large typeface. Above the beginning of the poem is a graphic depicting Ovid presumably composing his poem. (The picture is anachronistic: it shows Ovid writing in a codex or paged book, when he would have been using a papyrus roll.) Above the graphic there is a summary of the poem by Lactantius Placidus. The commentary by the Renaissance humanist Raphael Regius surrounds the text. Regius's typeface is smaller than the typeface of Ovid, but there is still much more space devoted to the commentary than to the poem itself.

This complex page layout tended to disappear in what we might call the industrial age of printing (1800-1950). In the nineteenth century classical commentaries were still placed as notes at the bottom of the page. But most books just presented one text in a series of paragraphs. This trend continued in the twentieth century, when notes tended to be banished to the back of the book. The space of a modern printed book is quite uniform. However, the differentiated space of this sixteenth-century commentary is very informative. Regius's comments upon specific words and phrases are located conveniently near Ovid's text. The reader can move easily from text to commentary and back. Each textual layer conveys a different kind of information, and each requires a different kind of reading or interpretive methodology.

The editions of texts like Ovid's Metamorphoses offered their contemporary reader a sense of control over the text that came from the accessible arrangement of information. Such editions offer us today a significant precursor to a new electronic typography. Chris Neuwirth and David Kaufer at Carnegie Mellon University have in fact directly applied the lessons of the medieval and

Renaissance page layout in developing their collaborative editing environment called Prep. In the Prep editor a writer's original text is placed in one column, and then various comments and annotations are located in columns to the right of the original. The editor maintains the spacing of each column so that all the comments remain parallel to the original paragraph to which they refer. [Kaufer92]

P. OVIDII NASONIS
METAMORPHOSEON
LIBER PRIMVS.

ARGVMENTVM LACTANTII PLACIDI.

Chaos, uti Heſiodus indicat in uolumine, quod deorum originem continet, fuit mutua rerum confuſio, quæ poſtea in ſuas ſpecies diſtincta, & diſtributa eſt.; ita ut leuiſſimum corporum, ęther igneus, & hunc infra aer frigidus, ceteraq; ſidera ſublimem partem peterent: per quæ ſolis ſplendor ac lumen uagaretur, grauiſſimum autem, humus, liquorq; in ima parte ſubſiderent.

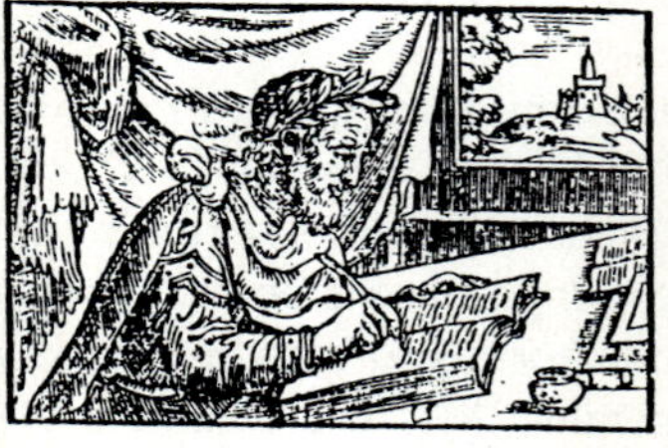

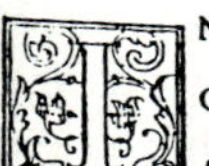

N noua fert animus mutatas dicere formas
Corpora. dij cœptis (nam uos mutaſtis & illas)
Aſpirate meis; primaque ab origine mundi
Ad mea perpetuum deducite tempora carmen.
Ante mare & terras, &, quod tegit omnia, cælum,

APH. N NOVA fert animus} conſueuerunt Heroici poetę in principiis ſtatim operum ſuorū proponere primum, quibus de rebus ſint in toto opere tractaturi, deinde inuocare, tertio loco narrare. quanquam Gręci ferè propoſitionem cū inuocatione coniungant. Eam conſuetudinem Ouid. quoq; in huius operis initio ſeruat. nam & breuiſſime ea, de quibus eſt ſcripturus, proponit; & deos, ut ſibi adeſſe uelint, rogat, & narrationem ab ipſo mundi primordio orditur. {In noua} eſt, inquit, mihi animus deſcribendi mutationes corporum in nouas figuras. Hac autem præpoſitione, quæ ſummam eorum continet, quæ in toto opere tractantur, & dociles & attenti lectores efficiuntur. {Fert animus} cupit. nam ferre inter alia ſignificata, eſt etiam cupere. {Mutatas formas} hoc eſt, corpora in nouas formas figurasq; mutata. eſt enim hypallage, poetis frequentiſſima. Eleganter aūt operis inſcriptionem expreſſit poeta. nam Metamorphoſis transformatio, ac formæ mutatio interpretatur. {Dii cœptis} deos inuocat, qui earūm mutationum auctores fuerunt, ut ſibi ita fauere uelint, ut quæ a principio mundi uſq; ad ſua tempora factæ ſunt mutationes, perpetuo carmine complecti poſſit. {Nam uos mutaſtis & illas} parentheſis eſt, cauſſam inuocationis continens. cum enim dii huiuſmodi mutationem fuerint auctores, facile eas memoriæ ſcribentis ſuppeditare poſſunt. Eſt autem ordo. Nam & uos mutaſtis illas. ac ſi diceret, uos, & non alii, fuiſtis auctores huiuſmodi transformationum. eſt enim emphaſis, qua plura innuuntur, quàm exprimantur. Minime uero imperitorum quorundam expoſitio eſt admittenda, putantium deos in uarias figuras eſſe mutatos, a poeta ſignificari, eoq; ſic eſſe ordinandum: Nam uos mutaſtis & illas. quo quidem modo ſenſus ex eleganti inſulſus efficeretur. periret enim illa emphaſis pulchra, quæ per copulam, Et, aperte demonſtratur. ſed huiuſmodi acuti ſenſus ab iſtis detractoribus ſtolidis, ingenioq; carentibus non percipiuntur. Hac autem expoſitione omnes, non deorum ſolum, ſed aliarum quoq; rerum tranſmutationes comprehenduntur. {Aſpirate} ſpiritum ac fauorem immittite. Eſt autem a uentis ſumpta translatio, qui dum nauiū uela implent, aſpirare proprie dicuntur. Virg. Aſpirat primo fortuna labori.

{Primaq; ab origine mundi} a prima mūdi creatione & conſtitutione. ſic autem a prima origine accipiendum eſt, non quod ſecunda fuerit, ſed a prima originis parte, ut dicimus in prima platea, in prima parte plateæ. nam a Chao ſumit exordiū, quod in quattuor, ait, fuiſſe transformatum elementa. Platonem uero, ac Stoicos ſequitur, qui ſentiunt mundum initium habuiſſe, a Deoq; genitū fuiſſe: quod Ariſt. negat: Mundus autem eſt (ut ait Poſidonius in Meteoris) qui conſtat ex cælo & terra, & terrenis cæleſtibusq; naturis: ſiue qui conſtat ex diis & hominibus, iisq; rebus, quæ horū gratia conditę ſunt. Ab ornatu uero tam latini mundum, quam Græci κόσμον appellant: ut Plin. ait. {Ad mea} uſque ad mea tempora. nā præpoſitio, uſq;, cum facile ſubintelligatur, eleganter in ſoluta quoque oratione, non ſolum in carmine, ſolet prætermitti. {Deducite} producite, protrahite. proprie autem (ut inquit Fabius) deduci carmina dicuntur, cum ſcribuntur. {Perpetuū} continuum, ſic ut nulla tranſmutatio prætermittatur, alteraq; alteri concinne, apteq; connectatur. id quod facile a diis impetrarat poeta. ita nanq; fabulam fabulæ annectit, ut una ex alia naſci uideatur. Sed quidam non minus inſulſus quam temerarius, quarundam ineptiarum interpoſitione ea in multis exemplaribus ſeparare conatus eſt, quæ deorū benignitate tam eleganter fuerant copulata. Id uero flagitium, quo totū opus inquinabatur, in primis curaui tollendum. {Ante mare & terras} hæc eſt narratio, quam a prima mundi origine poeta ſic repetit, ut deſcribat primam omnium mutationem. nam ex Heſiodi ſententia, quem potiſſimum hoc loco ſequitur Ouidius, primum omnium fuiſſe Chaos ait, hoc eſt quandam rerum omnium ſine ulla forma confuſionem, quæ materia prima a phyſicis uocatur. ex qua primum elementa quattuor, ac totum mundum effectum eſſe ait, cum antea nihil foret diſtinctum; ſed omnia ita eſſent confuſa, ut neque terra ab aere, neque aer ab aquis, neque aquæ ab æthere ſeparatæ eſſent. Primum itaq; deſcribit Ouidius Chaos ipſum: deinde narrat quemadmodum in quattuor elementa, ætherem, aerem, aquam, terram fuit cōmutatum, ſicq; diſcretum, ut æther ſummum locum propter leuitatem apprehenderit, proximum aer, aqua tertium, in infimum terra propter grauitatem detruſa fuerit,

prima origo mūdi.

A [Verſus

[Figure 1: Illustration of Humanist commentary (Raphael Regius)]

2. The Integration of Word and Image in Earlier Printing Technology

The illustration on the page of Ovid's poem indicates another dimension to early print technology. In the manuscript technology of the Middles Ages, there had been a great tradition of illumination: decorating letters of the text with elaborate abstract or figural designs. The earliest printed books used woodcuts to reproduce graphics; in the sixteenth century, copper engraving replaced woodcuts and allowed more precise and elaborate illustrations. With the improvement of printing technologies, the sixteenth century witnessed an explosion of graphic experimentation. These engravings could be decorative, or they could convey significant technical information (in books on anatomy and biology, in books containing maps, in technical manuals describing machinery, and so on). Graphics were also used to organize material and provide the reader with easy visual access to the subject matter. For a text such as Ovid's Metamorphoses, a large illustration at the beginning of a chapter functioned as a plan that could remind the reader of the narrative structure of the book; the picture could also reiterate the moral significance of individual passages.

In describing complex technical devices, a graphic could convey information more effectively than words, in particular because sixteenth writers had not yet developed a technical vocabulary in their own vernacular languages. Agostino Ramelli's (1588) illustration of a pulley system provides a good example. (See figure 2.)

Through detailed illustrations such as the one above, readers were able to grasp the relation between the parts of the machine and conceive how the parts fit together to achieve a specific purpose. In effect, illustrations such as this created a kind of short–hand that made scientists and technologists reluctant to depend only on written accounts ordinary language. Ramelli's illustration is clear and cogent, but the accompanying description is not [Ramelli1588, 1987]:

The mechanism of this next machine is most powerful for pulling and moving all kinds of very heavy weights. For when a man turns screw A with the crank, he thus turns worm gear B which has on the lower part of its shaft a toothed wheel marked H, and with this it turns the other two wheels on either side marked I K, together with the two drums L M set on their shafts. These drums wrap around themselves the end of the ropes that pass over the pulleys of the two tackles N O which are attached to the weight.[...]Like the drums marked L M, and at the same time, the other drums likewise wrap around themselves the other two ends of the ropes that are wound around the aforesaid pulleys and turning with these movements pull the weight with great ease, but also with the help given by the rollers which support it and are on the beams that exert force against the machine which pulls the weight, as is clearly understood by studying the drawing.

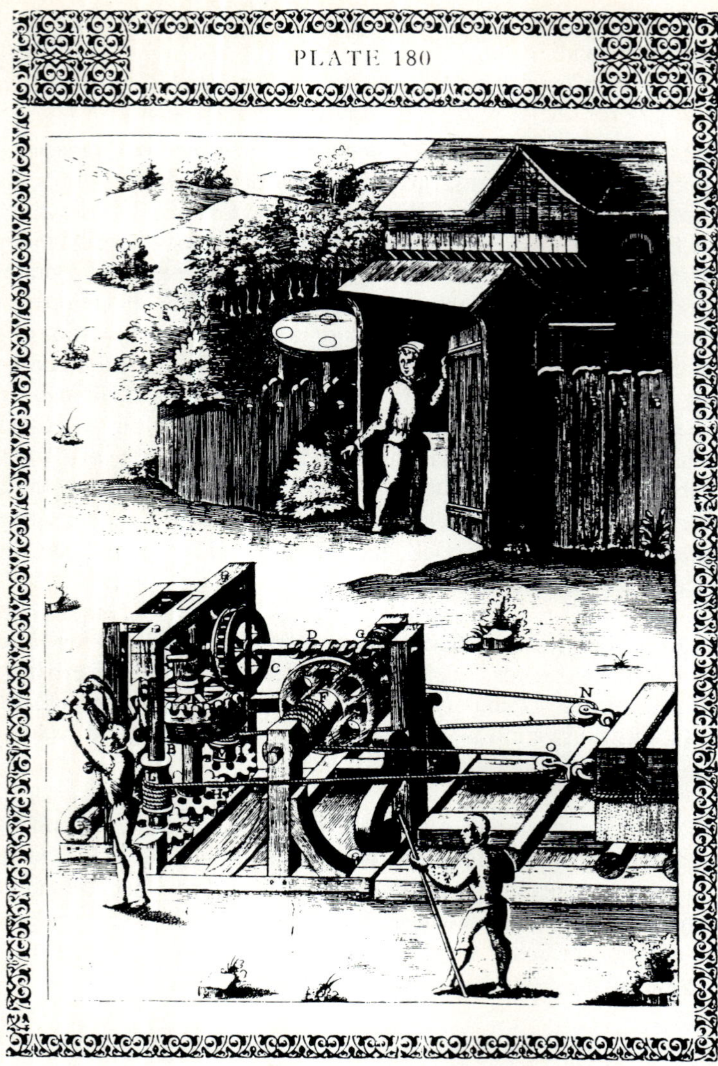

[Figure 2: Illustration of Gear and Pulley System]

Ramelli's text shows the phenomenon of doubling. He says things twice, once with a graphic and once in prose. It is as if the prose were trying to catch up to the graphic. One of the most developed Renaissance interpretive practices, allegory, may also be seen as doubling the written text with a graphic: the meaning of one medium becomes reinforced by the meaning of the other. Such doubling reminds us that the sixteenth- and seventeenth–century reader or observer expected that meaning or understanding would be supported by multiple registers. The multiple registers could be different kinds of verbal text, such as Regius's text, summary, and commentary for Ovid's Metamorphoses. But the multiple registers could also be different modes or media, such as Ramelli's combination of text and graphics.

Another and more elaborate example of the use of multiple modes is found in Michael Maier's Atalanta Fugiens (1618). (See figure 3.) Here Maier expects his reader to integrate graphic, texts, and even sound [Maier1618].

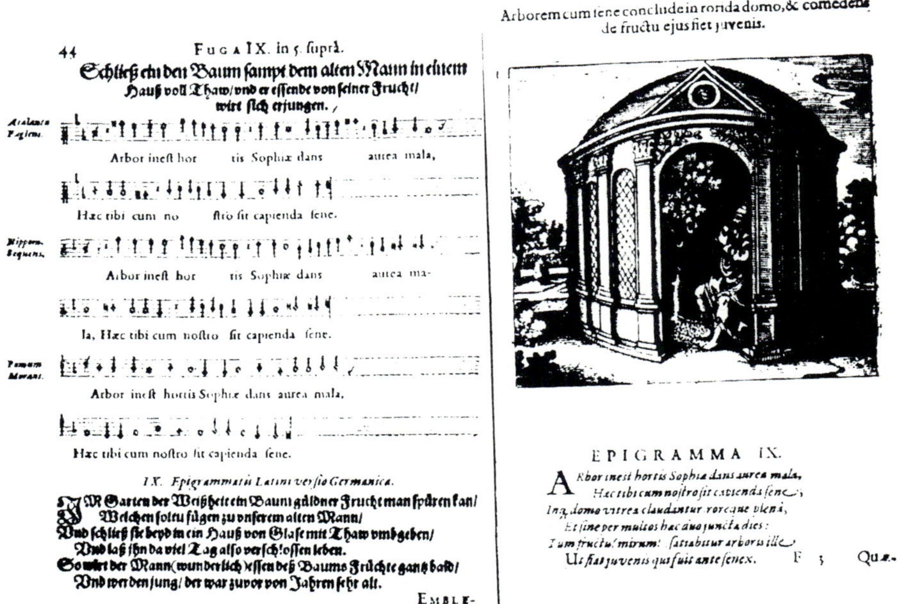
44 FUGA IX. in 5. suprà.

Schliess ein den Baum sampt dem alten Mann in einem Hauss voll Thaw/ und er essende von seiner Frucht/ wirt sich erjungen.

Atalanta Fugiens.

Arbor inest hor tis Sophiæ dans aurea mala,

Hæc tibi cum no stro sit capienda sene.

Hippom. Sequens.

Arbor inest hor tis Sophiæ dans aurea ma-

la, Hæc tibi cum nostro sit capienda sene.

Pomum Morans.

Arbor inest hortis Sophiæ dans aurea mala,

Hæc tibi cum nostro sit capienda sene.

IX. Epigrammatis Latini versio Germanica.

IM Garten der Weissheit ein Baum güldner Frucht man spüren kan/
Welchen soltu fügen zu unserem alten Mann/
Und schliess sie beyd in ein Hauss von Glase mit Thaw umbgeben/
Und lass ihn da viel Tag also verschlossen leben.
So wirt der Mann (wunderlich) essen dess Baums Früchte gantz bald/
Und werden jung/ der war zuvor von Jahren sehr alt.

EMBLE-

Arborem cum sene conclude in rorida domo, & comedens de fructu ejus fiet juvenis.

EPIGRAMMA IX.

ARbor inest hortis Sophiæ dans aurea mala,
Hæc tibi cum nostro sit capienda sene,
Inque domo vitrea claudantur roreque plena,
Et sine per multos hæc duo juncta dies:
Tum fructu (mirum!) satiabitur arboris ille,
Ut fiat juvenis qui fuit ante senex.

F 3 Quæ-

[Figure 3: Illustration of "Multimedia" Text]

This is truly a printed version of multimedia. By placing musical notation on the same pages with words and graphics, Maier is creating a multimedia event. The problem of course is that the media, particularly the music, are not self-activating. The reader must activate the text by reading the words, examining the graphics, and presumably playing and singing the music. This static combination of media is as far as the printed book could go in the direction of integration. The technology of printing achieved this level of integration as early as the seventeenth century. And, if anything, the tendency to integrate declined in the printing of the nineteenth and twentieth centuries.

3. Text and Graphics in the Electronic Writing Space

These examples from the period of craft printing can provide us with a new perspective on the development of multimedia today. In that early period of printing, illustrations of technical ideas were sometimes more sophisticated than prose descriptions. We have seen how authors would repeat in prose what the graphic illustrated. The new writing space of the computer also offers possibilities for the doubling of text and graphics. A graphic may reinforce the meaning of a verbal text or vice versa. Text and graphics may interact in more complicated ways, too. This interaction has not been fully appreciated in the computer medium, perhaps because the late age of industrial printing did not exploit graphic doubling as did the earlier period of craft printing. And it is this late age of printing that directly influenced the development of word processing in the 1970s and 1980s. The task of the craft printers was both to develop an appropriate space for the written word and to explore how to combine alphabetic text with illustrations and diagrams. Developers of multimedia now face a similar task in defining an electronic space that integrates words, graphics, sound, and video.

A number of approaches are possible. Perhaps the most obvious is to deploy text in and around the graphics, as we now do with captions in printed books. This is already done, for example, with menus and labels in the standard desktop metaphor. Various objects on the desktop (file, directories, and applications) carry their textual name around with them. Techniques of deploying text in this fashion can be learned from traditional graphic design and illustration. But even here new questions arise when we add motion. With animated graphics and video, the images change over time, and so certain kinds of labels for these sequences of images also need to be time-dependent, appearing when the image is appropriate and disappearing later in the sequence. A model here, interestingly enough, could be subtitles in films, which change to reflect the current spoken dialogue.

However, there are other, more significant ways in which the symbolic role (ordinarily played by language) and the visual role (played graphics and video) can be integrated. In some multimedia applications, the graphic elements themselves may be assigned a symbolic role: that is, they may become textual elements with a symbolic meaning. We can call this the "textualizing of the graphic space." Such textualizing is in fact already a well-established technique in the field of scientific visualization. In such applications scientists are permitted to see their data in a visually enhanced space. The space is symbolic in the sense that it is generated by setting up a coded relationship between graphic elements (such as size, color, and shape) and the (usually numerical) data.

Scientific visualization shows how one can construct a symbolic space out of numerical data. But we wish here to focus attention on verbal text rather than numbers. We propose as a research question whether verbal text could also be deployed effectively in a symbolic space-either in some form of projected 3D graphics or in Virtual Reality. In this way the text would not serve merely to label objects; it would instead be used to communicate verbal ideas, as it does now in the two-dimensional space of the printed page. A three-dimensional symbolic space could be laid out to suit the text, which might appear floating in space or attached to walls, blocks, or other objects. The goal would be to use visual cues to aid the reader/user in locating and assimilating information. We call this proposal (which is the converse of scientific visualization) "spatializing the text."

4. Spatializing the Text

There is some previous work from which we can draw for the setting out of verbal text in a graphic space. Several recent hypertext systems provide concept maps for editing or browsing; these maps are graphical representations of the structure of texts and links in the hypertext. One system that provides concept maps is Storyspace, an environment for creating and delivering small and medium-sized hypertexts.[Joyce91] Storyspace offers a graphic representation, in which nodes are shown as boxes and links as arrows. (See figure 4.) The map is updated to reflect structural changes as they occur, and the author can make such changes on the map itself, by grabbing and moving the boxes. Spatial relationships in Storyspace are significant: nodes can be clustered to indicate conceptual relationships.

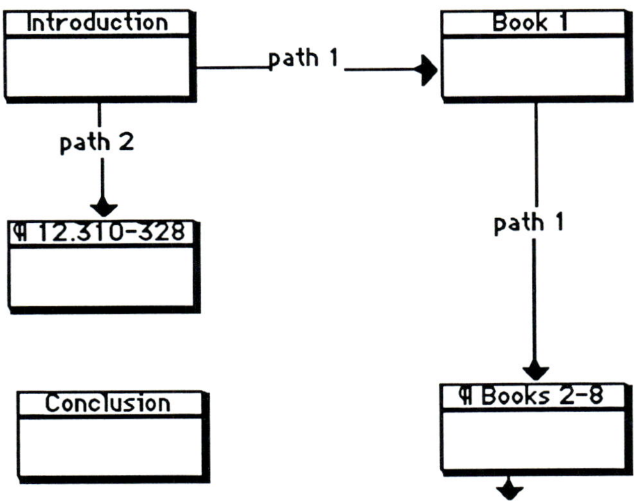

[Figure 4: Concept map in Storyspace]

Other systems have employed a variety of techniques for visualizing the semantics of the hypertext. Jerker Andersson describes a system for hypertextual mapping elsewhere in this volume. We can also point to Sepia, developed at the Integrated Publication and Information Systems Institute in Darmstadt.[Streitz89; Thüring91] There is the MacWeb System developed by Jocelyn and Marc Nanard. [Nanard91] There is also Acquanet, where complex semantic relationships among the elements are expressed through spatial layout. In all these systems, alphabetic text (the names and, in some cases, even the contents of the cells) may be integrated into the graphic space.

If two-dimensional concept maps are a proven tool, it is plausible that a three-dimensional representation will make the structure clearer and easier to edit and browse. There has already been some work in this area. Semnet developed at MCC in the mid 1980s provided three-dimensional visualizations of a semantic net.[Fairchild88] More recently, researchers at Xerox Parc have created the 3D/Rooms interface, in which hierarchies of information are presented as tree structures in three dimensions called "cone trees." The cones can be rotated to facilitate viewing [Card91, Robertson91]. A three-dimensional information browser is also being developed by Hemmje at IPSI in Darmstadt. [Hemmje93] These systems suggest that textual information can be searched for and digested effectively in three dimensions. Although the 3D/Rooms and the IPSI systems are not hypertexts with arbitrary links, it also seems likely that a third dimension would help in untangling the spaghetti that sometimes results from the intersection of many links in a two-dimensional hypertextual concept map. In a three-dimensional view, the user could change his or her perspective, so that fewer links would have to intersect.

5. The Virtual Book

Arranging text in three dimensions calls for a new typography. The typography of current printed books is generally limited to a few simple visual structures. Paragraphs and headings convey local organization of the page or the opening. Larger structures are conveyed by the table of contents and indices, which are then mapped to the linear order of the pages. The design of a magazine or newspaper page makes more creative use of its visual space. The reader's eye is invited to move around the page and focus upon interesting material. In fact, contemporary magazines are really the successors of the examples of craft printing that we discussed earlier. For example, many magazines and newspapers make use of the techniques of integration (locating text in and around graphics) and doubling (using a graphic to restate the verbal text or vice versa). However, a printed magazine is still a layout only in two dimensions. Adding a third dimension opens a new range of typographic possibilities. This new place in which to locate text might be called a "virtual book." It remains an open research question whether such a spatial arrangement will in fact clarify structure and make it easier to navigate through textual information. But again, it seems plausible that it would, as the following example suggests.

A traditional table of contents in a printed book shows the topics in serial order together with their appropriate page numbers. (See figure 5.) To make a three-dimensional version, we could create a block for each topic and array the topics in space. (See figure 6.) This spatial arrangement provides more information in at least two ways. First, clusters of pages (or other units) are visible at a distance, giving the user a sense of the overall structure. This sense of structure is refined as the user moves closer to particular areas of the text. Second, at certain distances and perspectives, the user will be able to see the text of several pages at once. Portions of text on those pages or units may be in large typeface and will be visible at a greater distance. As the user moves closer, more of the text becomes legible.

Georgia Institute of Technology

••••••••••••••••••••••••••••

General Information...6
Information for Undergraduate Students.......................................22
Information for Graduate Students.......................................34
Financial Information.......................................44
Curricula and Courses of Instruction.......................................53
College of Architecture.......................................55
College of Computing.......................................81
College of Engineering.......................................93
Ivan Allen College of Management.......................................205
College of Sciences.......................................272
Rules and Regulations.......................................326
Administration, Faculty, Staff.......................................342
Campus Map.......................................371
Index.......................................373

[Figure 5: Conventional table of contents]

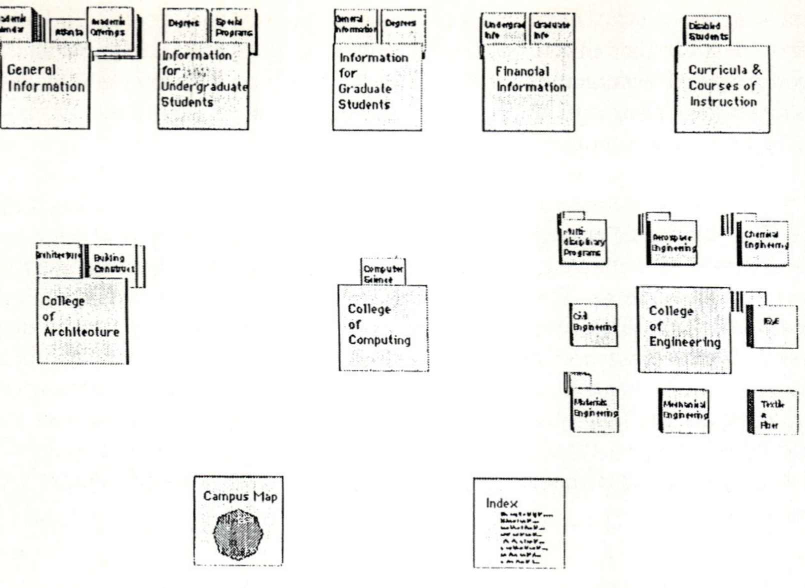

[Figure 6: Spatial layout of table of contents in Figure 5.]

In our example, the traditional layout of the table of contents gives no visual prominence to the fact that one of the sections ("College of Engineering") is much longer and more detailed than the others. The user would have to look closely at the page numbers to notice the importance of the one section. However, the spatial representation makes the prominence of this section clear at a glance, because of the large number of unit markers clustering around the section.

This is only one way in which a third dimension might be added to the traditional hierarchical or linear layouts found in printed texts. Our sample space resembles a hypertextual concept map without the links, and certainly hypertextual links (as arrows) could be drawn all through this space. Color, shape, and size could also be used to discriminate among the units in a three-dimensional space. Figure 6 uses different sizes to indicate the importance of a particular block. Different colors might also indicate whether a textual block had recently been modified. Shapes could indicate different types of text. All of these techniques have already been employed in or suggested for two-dimensional hypertextual concept maps.

On the other hand, the spatialization of the text might proceed in a direction very different from that of the abstract concept maps of hypertext systems. For example, an architectural metaphor might prove effective for conveying structure. Human beings have a great deal of experience in understanding and navigating in built environments: houses, buildings, neighborhoods, and cities. This experience of place could be given symbolic significance. For example, chapters in a book might be laid out as rooms on an architectural surface, and the architecture of the whole layout and of each room might be used to convey structure. (See figure 7.) In the center of the layout, an information kiosk (not shown here) would contain summary information and the location of each chapter. Further summary information would be located at the entrance to each room, and within each room the walls themselves would present the text in detail.

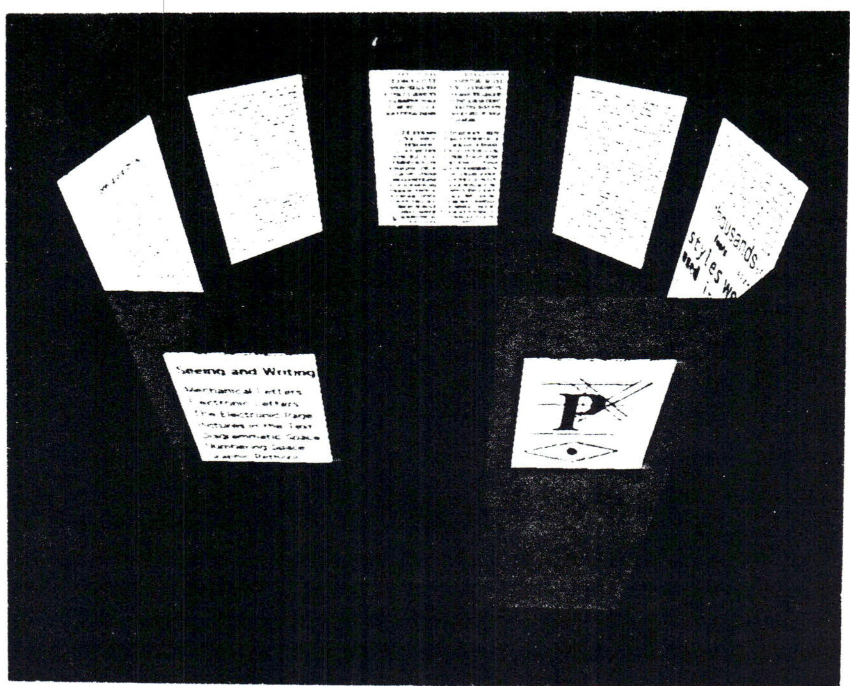

[Figure 7]

This metaphor too is being explored at the Zentrum für Graphische Datenverarbeitung in Darmstadt: multimedia information is being represented as located inside rooms of a house. [Hübner93] There is also a much earlier forerunner–the ancient mnemonic system called the "art of memory," used in the ancient world and in the Middle Ages. An ancient orator remembered the points of a speech by placing vivid images at various locations in a well-known building; he later recalled the points by mentally traversing the building as he spoke. [Yates66]

6. Technical Limits to Spatialization

Current hardware limits what can be done with the spatialization of text. The limitations are particularly obvious for displaying text in Virtual Reality. Head-mounted displays often do not give adequate resolution for reading text. For example, a prototype system for spatializing text in VR has been constructed in the Graphics, Visualization, and Usability Center at the Georgia Institute of Technology. The system uses the conventionally available equipment, including a Virtual Research head-mounted display and a Silicon Graphics Indigo Elan workstation [Verlinden93]. Texts in this system can be created either by drawing individual letters graphically by algorithm or by scanning pages of text and placing these scanned images in the space through texture mapping. This system is useful for experiments–it produced Figure 3 above–but it is not adequate for long reading sessions. However, texture mapping works well when displayed on higher resolution screens rather than in the helmet. And even the resolution of head-mounted displays should continue to improve. So as we develop new typographies for 3D and Virtual Reality space, we can anticipate improvements in the hardware to accommodate these developments.

7. Spatial Metaphors

It seems unlikely that a house or other conventional architecture will provide the best spatial metaphor. Our point is rather that work needs to be done to discover which spatial metaphors might be most effective. The human sense of being oriented in space is a powerful tool by which we organize information. We sometimes remember a passage in printed books merely on the basis of its position on a particular page. We place books and papers on our desk and bookshelves and rely on a sense of place to find them again. We learn to use a library by becoming acquainted with the arrangement of books and materials on various floors. The two-dimensional desktop metaphor already proves the effectiveness of the spatial arrangement of text in an computer interface. A sense of spatial organization should be even easier to engender in a three-dimensional environment.

Research on the spatialization of text can draw upon a wide variety of disciplines–some closely allied to computer science and others traditionally quite distant. As we argued in the first half of this paper, the history of typography and graphic design offers lessons that may be used in designing a new kind of virtual book. Contemporary graphic design also has much to say about combining text and images in two dimensions. For spatial metaphors, traditional architecture can help. When architects design buildings and built environments, they pay careful attention to the ways in which a human user will move through the space and will understand the structure of the environment as he or she moves. There is a related literature in perceptual psychology, on the subject of way-finding in a neighborhood, city, or any natural or synthetic environment. Finally, as we have mentioned, work on spatial layout and navigation of text can draw on existing work in hypertextual mapping and navigation.

Applications for three-dimensional text would certainly include textual and multimedia databases. The conceptual structure of a large textual database could be mapped out in three dimensions so that the user could remain oriented as he or she conducted a query. The same technique could be applied to databases that include pictures or other media. In three-dimensional space a picture or even a video could be shown on a wall together with text. Spatialization should aid in the visualization of any kind of hypertextual information. In general this technique may be a partial solution to the problem of being "lost in hyperspace." A user is lost, when he or she can no longer relate the current information to the hypertext as a whole. But if the user is surrounded by a spatial version of the hypertextual structure, then visual cues can help to maintain a sense of the whole as the user moves.

Representing text in three dimensions is therefore both a new and a traditional idea. It is new in the sense that such representations are only possible with the advent of powerful personal computers and workstations and three-dimensional graphics. It is traditional in that it draws upon a whole history of verbal-visual communication in printed books and early writing technologies.

References

[2992] ISO/IEC JTC1/SC 29. Coded Representation of Multimedia and Hypermedia Information Objects, Part 1: Base Notation - Working Document S.6. ISO/IEC, October 1992.

[Beninger78] James R. Beninger and Dorothy L. Robyn, Quantitative Graphics in Statistics: A Brief History, American Statistician, 32, (1978), 1-11.

[Calandri1491] Filippo Calandri, Aritmetica (1491), ff. [?]

[Card91] S. K. Card, Robertson G. G., and Macinlay, J. D. The Information

Visualizer, An Information Workspace. Proceedings of CHI '91 (New Orleans, 1991), New York: ACM, pp. 181-188.

[Eisenstein79] Elizabeth L. Eisenstein, The Printing Press as an Agent of Change 2 vols. (Cambridge: Cambridge Univ. Press, 1979)

[Fairchild88] K.M. Fairchild, Poltrock, S. E., & Furnas, G. W. SemNet: Three-dimensional Graphic Representation of Large Knowledge Bases. In Cognitive Science and its Application for Human-Computer Interface, R. Guindon (ed.). Hillsdale, New Jersey: Lawrence Erlbaum, 1988.

[Galileo1611] Discoveries and Opinions of Galileo, ed. Stillman Drake (New York: Doubleday Anchor, 1957), 35.

[Hemmje88] M. A. Hemmje, 3D Based User Interface for Information Retrieval Systems, paper submitted to SIGIR '93, Pittsburgh, June 27, 1993.

[Hübner93] W. Hübner, V. Burrill, and K. Väänänen, Advanced User Interfaces for 3D and Multimedia Interaction. In Multimedia: System Architectures and Applications, J. Encarnaçâo and J. Foley (eds.). Darmstadt, Germany: Zentrum für Graphische Datenverarbeitung, 1993.

[HyT92] ISO/IEC IS 10744: Information Technology - Hypermedia/Time-Based Structuring Language (HyTime). ISO/IEC, 1992.

[Joyce91] Michael Joyce. Storyspace as a hypertext system for writers and readers of varying ability. Hypertext '91 Proceedings, San Antonio, Texas, (15-18 December, 1991), 381-388.

[Kaufer92] David S. Kaufer, Christine M. Neuwirth, Ravinder Chandhok, and James H. Morris, Writing: A Retrospective on Computer-Support for Open-Ended Design Tasks. In Learning to Design, Designing to Learn (D. Ferguson, D. Balestri and S. Ehrmann, eds.), (New York, Taylor and Francis, 1992), pp. 119-137.

[Laurel91] Brenda Laurel, Computers as Theatre (Reading, Mass.: Addison-Wesley, 1991).

[Maier1618] Michael Maier, Atalanta Fugiens (Frankfort, 1618),

[Marshall91] Catherine C. Marshall, Frank G. Halasz, Russell A. Rogers, and William C. Janssen Jr., Aquanet: A Hypertext Tool to Hold Your Knowledge in Place, Hypertext '91 Proceedings, San Antonio, Texas, (15-18 December, 1991), 261-275.

[Nanard91] Jocelyn Nanard and Mark Nanard, Using Structured Types to Incorporate Knowledge in Hypertexts, Hypertext '91 Proceedings, San Antonio, Texas, (15-18 December, 1991), 329-344.

[ODA89] ISO/IEC IS 8613: Information Processing - Text and Office Systems - Office Document Architecture (ODA) and Interchange Format (ODIF) ISO/IEC, 1989.

[Ramelli1588, 1987] Agostino Ramelli, Diverse et Artificiose Machine (Lyon, 1588). I have used the reprint of Ramelli found in The Various Machines of Agostino Ramelli, tran. Martha Teach Gnudi with technical annotations by Eugene S. Ferguson (New York: Dover Publications, Inc., 1987).

[Ramelli, 1987] The Various Machines of Agostino Ramelli, 470.

[Regius1565] Raphael Regius, Metamorphoseon (Venice, 1565), 1.

[Robertson91] G. G. Robertson, Jock D. Macinlay, S. K. Card, Cone Trees: Animated 3D Visualizations of Hierarchical Information. Proceedings of CHI '91 (New Orleans, April,1991). New York: ACM, 1991.

[Streitz89] Norbert Strietz, J. Hannemann, M. Thüring, From Ideas and Arguments to Hyperdocuments: Travelling Through Activity Spaces, Proceedings Hypertext '89, 1989.

[Thüring91] Manfred Thüring, Jörg M. Haake, Jörg Hannemann, What's Eliza Doing in the Chinese Room? Incoherent Hyperdocuments and How to Avoid Them, Hypertext '91 Proceedings, San Antonio, Texas, (15-18 December, 1991), 161-178.

[Verlinden93] Jouke C. Verlinden, Jay David Bolter, Charles van der Mast, "The World Processor: An Interface for Textual Display and Manipulation in Virtual Reality." Graphic, Visualization, and Usability Center, Georgia Institute of Technology, Technical Report #1993.

[Yates66] Frances A. Yates, The Art of Memory. Chicago, University of Chicago Press, 1966.] Frances A. Yates, The Art of Memory. Chicago, University of Chicago Press, 1966.

Printing: Mercedesdruck, Berlin
Binding: Buchbinderei Lüderitz & Bauer, Berlin